YOUR PRECIOUS SIGHT

An Optometrist's Most Memorable Cases

Eichin Chang-Lim, O.D.

YOUR PRECIOUS SIGHT
Copyright © 2019 Eichin Chang-Lim, O.D.

All rights reserved.

No part of this publication may be reproduced, transmitted, or distributed by any person or entity (including, but not confined to, Google, Amazon or similar and related organizations), in any form or by any means, electronic or mechanical, including photocopy, recording, scanning or any information storage and retrieval system, without permission in writing from the author.

Medical and Professional Disclaimer:

The people and situations mentioned in this book are based on real patients and cases. However, in order to abide by the principles of protecting patients' privacy and confidentiality, the names and many of the specifications have been adjusted and fictionalized. Any similarities to real people, living or dead, are unintentional and entirely coincidental.

The author does not recommend or endorse any sites or products or advertisements presented in this book or associated with any sites or links. The author has no financial affiliation or financial interest with any products presented or associated with any sites or links mentioned or referenced in this book. All the sites and links are provided merely as references for readers. The author has made her best effort to ensure the accuracy and authenticity of the information; however, due to the complexity and rapid advances in the medical field and healthcare, the author cannot be held accountable or assume liability for any information that is outdated or inaccurate. This book and any reference sites or links or advertisements are not a substitute for ocular or healthcare advice. If you have any questions or concerns about your or your family's health, you should always contact your own eye doctor or other healthcare professional.

www.eichinchanglim.com

Edited by Susan Hughes
Formatted by The Book Khaleesi

10 9 8 7 6 5 4 3 2 1

CONTENTS

Other Books by Eichin Chang-Lim vii

Preface xi

Diagram of the Eye xv

What is a Dilated Fundus Examination (DFE)? xvii

Chapter 1 1

    The Stories of Amblyopia (Lazy Eyes) and Strabismus (Crossed Eyes)

Chapter 2 16

    The Stories of Color Deficiency

Chapter 3 25

    When is the Right Age to Introduce Contact Lenses to Youngsters?

Chapter 4 37

    The Stories of Conjunctivitis (Red Eye/Pink Eye)

Chapter 5 47

    The Stories of Eye Allergies

Chapter 6 55

    The Stories of Retinitis Pigmentosa

Chapter 7 65

    The Stories of Computer Glasses, Sports and

Work Safety, and Sun Protection

Chapter 8 .... **84**

The Stories of Refractive Surgeries

Chapter 9 .... **95**

The Stories of Multiple Sclerosis

Chapter 10 .... **105**

The Stories of Eye Twitching, Central Serous Retinopathy, and Hysterical Blindness

Chapter 11 .... **117**

The Stories of How Substance Abuse and Smoking Affect the Eyes

Chapter 12 .... **126**

The Stories of Retinal Detachments (RD)

Chapter 13 .... **137**

The Stories about More than the Headaches, Double Vision, and Blurred Vision

Chapter 14 .... **150**

The Stories of Diabetic Patients

Chapter 15 .... **161**

The Stories of Needing Reader or Multifocal Lenses

Chapter 16 .... **169**

The Stories of Dry Eyes

Chapter 17 .... **181**

The Stories of Open-Angle Glaucoma (Silent Thief of Sight) and Acute Angle-Closure Glaucoma

Chapter 18 .... **195**

The Stories of Flashes of Light and Floaters

Chapter 19 .... **206**

The Stories of Age-Related Macular Degeneration (AMD)

Chapter 20 .... **217**

The Stories about Cataracts and Cataract Surgeries

Chapter 21 .... **227**

The Stories of Renewing Driver's Licenses and Safe Driving

Acknowledgments **239**

Three Kinds of Eye Care Professionals **243**

Glossary of Common Eye and Vision Conditions **245**

Valuable Resources **251**

References **253**

About the Author **263**

Other Books by Eichin Chang-Lim

The LoveLock

A Mother's Heart

Love: A Tangled Knot

Flipping

To *YOU* who are taking your eye care as seriously as I am

"Periodic eye and vision examinations are an important part of preventive health care. Many eye and vision problems have no obvious signs or symptoms, so you might not know a problem exists. Early diagnosis and treatment of eye and vision problems can help prevent vision loss."

~*American Optometric Association (AOA)*

"You might think your vision is in good shape or that your eyes are healthy, but visiting your eye care professional for a comprehensive dilated eye exam is the only way to be completely certain."

~*National Eye Institute (NEI)*

Preface

BEING BLIND IS one of the biggest fears for most humans. No one wants to live in the "dark!" Many times, my patients have asked me, "Doc, am I going blind?" I have all the empathy in the world for their anguish. I heard this question innumerable times during my formative years.

One winter morning, my father woke up and discovered he had abruptly lost his vision in his left eye. Eye care was not as sophisticated and advanced then, so the vision in that eye never returned. We were clueless as to why the light had turned off in that eye. Many years later, I checked his eyes and suspected that he'd had an acute retinal vein occlusion due to a history of eye injury. For years, he was afraid of opening his eyes upon awakening to discover that he had lost his vision in the other eye. It was like a gloomy cloud that hung over my family for as long as I could remember.

You might think that I'd always aimed to become an eye doctor; I wish I had a glorious story to share with you. However, that's not the case in reality. I came to this country to pursue my master's degree in microbiology. While busily applying to a PhD program and doing research in a hematology lab at the UCLA Medical Center, my boyfriend at the time—my husband now—expressed his passion and goal to become an optometrist. He invited me to apply to the optometry school with him. I did with hesitance. We were both accepted and enrolled in optometry school together.

Retrospectively, that is one of the best decisions I have made in my life. After decades of being in the eye care profession, the excitement and astonishment from examining patients' eyes and looking into their "windows to the soul" have never waned. The eye is such a marvelous organ. It's one of the smallest organs in the human body—the average size of an adult eyeball is approximately two-thirds the size of a ping pong ball—yet it controls the majority of our learning, thinking, and daily activities. Our eyes are like a small mirror, which reflects our entire body's systemic function.

I am writing this manuscript to share with you a few memorable cases from my thirty years as an eye care professional and to illustrate the value of a comprehensive eye examination. This book is not intended to be an eye care guide.

Since the human eye is such a delicate organ, there are hundreds and hundreds of known—and unknown—genetic and acquired disorders associated with it, and volumes of textbooks depict and study all of the ocular and vision anomalies, diagnoses, and treatments. My goal is to encourage you not to take your eyesight for granted.

In the meantime, I treasure all of my relationships with my patients, many of whom have become great friends. I want to express my gratitude to all who trust me, allow me to examine and look into their eyes, and generously share their stories with me. You have taught me so much about the beauty of the human soul and love demonstrated globally in the eyes of diverse people.

Last but not least, my immense thanks to my instructors, classmates, colleagues, and friends who have supported me and encouraged me to be a better optometrist in the profession of eye care.

Diagram of the Eye

https://nei.nih.gov/health/eyediagram

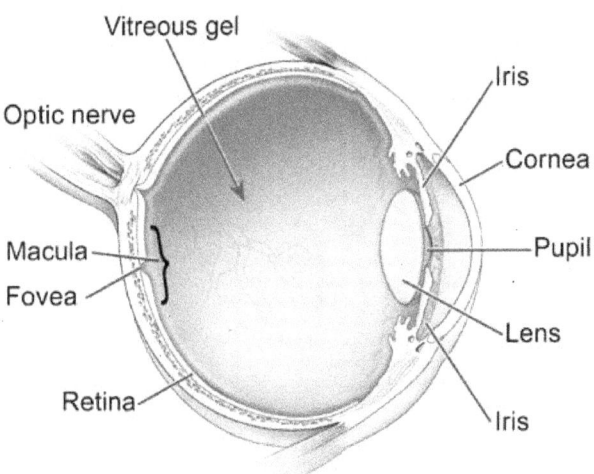

What is a Dilated Fundus Examination (DFE)?

THE FUNDUS OF the eye is the interior back surface of the eyeball. DFE is a procedure to check the fundus. Some practitioners may refer to it as a dilated retinal exam or dilated eye exam. The analogy that I applied to communicate with my patients about DFE is something like this: "For me, not dilating your eyes is like peeking into a room through a keyhole. With dilation, it's like opening the door to check every corner of the room."

DFE involves instilling dilating drops into the eyes. It usually takes about twenty to thirty minutes to take effect. People with darker eye color tend to have to wait longer for the eye to be fully dilated due to the amount of pigmentation in the iris (colored part of the eye).

How long the eyes will be dilated depends on the concentration and type of dilating agent. Your eye care professional can provide you the estimated time. When your eyes are dilated, you will have difficulty seeing close objects and be sensitive to bright light. You should avoid handling a vehicle and machinery.

DFE can detect early glaucoma, cataract, age-related macular degeneration, unusual fundus pigmentation (a precursor of eye cancer in some cases), peripheral retina thinning, other fundus abnormalities, and systemic eye-related diseases such as diabetic retinopathy or vascular changes caused by hypertension.

I recommend that you watch the Animation of Dilated Eye Exam from the National Eye Institute, National Institutes of Health (NIH) on YouTube.

Chapter 1

"I failed the school screening. My teacher said I might have a lazy eye."

The Stories of Amblyopia (Lazy Eyes) and Strabismus (Crossed Eyes)

"Lazy eye, or amblyopia, often occurs in people who have crossed eyes (misalignment) or a large difference in the degree of nearsightedness or farsightedness (or astigmatisms) between the two eyes."

~AOA

I WALKED INTO the exam room and was met by a crowd.

It was an amusing scene!

My exam room measured thirteen feet by

fourteen feet. In the far corner, a 60-gallon aquarium hosted a turtle and two fish. The other corner had two armchairs side by side and a rocking horse next to the chairs. An exam chair positioned three feet away from the back wall attached to some of the ophthalmic instruments and scope chargers, and a mirror was placed on the opposite wall to reflect the digital eye chart. My desk was a couple of feet beside the exam chair with a computer on it.

I saw three boys of various heights standing around the aquarium. A girl who appeared to be around four years old was rocking on the wooden horse. A young girl with a ponytail was perched in the exam chair. A younger lady was seated on one armchair with an infant; an older woman was seated on the other armchair and held a sleeping toddler.

"Who is Rosa?" I asked. The name on the exam form was Rosa PJ Mendosa-Gonsalez, six years old. The girl on the exam chair raised her hand, and the three older boys turned around, pointing at her simultaneously.

"Is there a special reason Rosa is here?" I asked the younger woman. She directed her gaze toward the tallest boy before I finished my

YOUR PRECIOUS SIGHT

question.

A conversation in Spanish ensued for at least three minutes between the two women and the two bigger boys. I have always loved to have a room filled with a family and observe their dynamic interactions. Finally, the younger woman, whom I realized was all of the kids' mother, extracted a wrinkled paper from a bag and handed it to me. It was a school vision screening report.

With the sweetest voice, little Rosa spoke up before her brothers had a chance to say anything. "I failed the school eye test. My teacher said I might have a lazy eye. My mom needs to bring me in to have an eye exam. The doctor needs to fill out this form. I need to bring it back to my teacher." I was glad she explained everything and was impressed by her articulation and confidence.

The screening exam report stated that the vision in her right eye was 20/30, and the left eye was 20/100. There was a question mark next to the last number. After looking at the auto-reflector printout—a computerized instrument that provides the approximate measurement of an eye that needs to be corrected with spectacles or contact lenses—of the pretest done by my assistant, I proceeded to the preliminary examinations eye muscle moments, confrontation visual field, and the anterior segment of her eyes.

I said to Rosa, "To check your eyes better, I need to put drops into your eyes. It will feel like water gets into your eyes when you go swimming in the pool. Can you tell your mother?" She quickly translated the message.

The mother consented.

The results revealed that her right eye was slightly farsighted, with minimal astigmatism; however, her left eye had 8 diopters of astigmatism. This meant her eyeball was shaped like an American football, causing the light rays to scatter in the back of the eye and making objects appear blurred. With the prescription, she obtained a pair of glasses via Medi-Cal, California's equivalent to Medicaid, to wear full time. She was also instructed to do pencil drawings, colorings, and watch TV with her left eye while patching the right eye for two hours a day. It was near Halloween, so she could ask her mom to get her an eye patch at Party City.

A year later, she returned without glasses. "I was holding my baby brother. He pulled my

YOUR PRECIOUS SIGHT

glasses off and broke them," she said with agony. I rechecked her prescription; her best correctable vision was 20/20 on the right eye and 20/60 on the left eye. Assuming an object is visible at sixty feet with 20/20 vision, that same object isn't clearly seen until it is at and within twenty feet with 20/60 vision.

"I did not do the eye patch every day like you told me," Rosa admitted.

Medi-Cal only allows one pair of glasses every two years; however, we were able to obtain an authorization to get her a replacement at that time.

Her maturity was beyond her age, and after discussing it with my practice partner, we decided to fit her with bitoric rigid gas-permeable contact lenses (RGP) when she was eight years old, with the funding contributed by the local Lion's Club. The bitoric RGP lenses would provide much sharper vision and less distortion than the spectacles on her left eye, for it rested right on the cornea, the clear front surface of the eye.

Note: Bitoric contact lenses are a type of gas-permeable contact lens with two different curvatures, one on the front surface and the other one on the back surface. Most of the time, it's prescribed when the corneal astigmatism is equal to or exceeds 2.50 diopters.

With these lenses and diligently patching her right eye to force the left eye to work harder, her best correctable vision was 20/20 (right) and 20/25+ (left) when she went to take her driver's license exam at age seventeen.

We all cheered her achievement when she was accepted at UCLA with a scholarship right after high school. There is no better reward for an eye doctor than seeing her patients strive and soar.

For vision like Rosa's, our goal was to give the patient total vision correction to wear full time, so that objects cast clear images on the retina, and the brain received the optimal stimulation. "Lazy eye," amblyopia in medical terms, is caused by blurred images on the retina and a lack of full stimulation of the brain. We patch the good eye to force the other eye to work harder in the hope that both eyes will reach an equally good correctable vision to achieve binocularity and depth perception eventually.

YOUR PRECIOUS SIGHT

Before departing from this section, let me share with you the following quote from NEI:

*"**Amblyopia** is the medical term used when the vision in one of the eyes is reduced because the eye and the brain are not working together properly. The eye itself looks normal, but it is not being used normally because the brain is favoring the other eye. This condition is also sometimes called lazy eye."*

~ * ~

*"**Strabismus**, also called crossed eyes, is when your eyes do not line up in the same direction when you focus on an object. A variety of conditions can cause strabismus."*

~ *NEI*

WE WERE AT the Vision Expo West in the Sands Convention Center, Las Vegas. After two hours of sitting in classes, visiting the exhibit hall, and hugging and talking with a few classmates I hadn't seen in a while, I sat near the waterfall in the atrium of the Venetian Hotel, doing what I always loved the most: people watching.

"Watch out. Stop running," a female voice screamed out.

Aww! In Taiwanese! I understand what she said! So familiar. So sweet.

I quickly turned toward the source of the voice. A woman ran after a child. She picked him up, held him, and sat him on the bench where I was. The mother scolded him gently, again in Taiwanese. I could not help but smile at her.

"Vacationing?" I asked her in Taiwanese. From there, we conversed in our mother tongue. I found out the boy, named Sean, was four years old.

"Would you mind taking a look at Sean's eyes? I think his eyes are crossed," the mother asked politely and hesitantly after she found out why I was in Vegas and what my profession was.

I consciously looked down at my ID, attached to a lanyard, which I had not removed.

Do an eye exam a few feet from the casino? Hmm.

YOUR PRECIOUS SIGHT

I searched the goody bag from one of the vendors in the exhibit hall and found a smiley sticker and an appropriately sized card to use for the cover test to check the eyes' alignment. I put the smiley on my left index finger.

"I can take a look, but it's not a real eye exam," I said to the mother, emphasizing the last part of the statement. My California license won't cover Nevada.

The mother coaxed Sean to turn toward me. His black, twinkly eyes were not aligned. I could tell right away.

"You are such a big boy. Let's play a game. Can you look at the sticker and hold your head still?" I hunkered down to his eye level, raised my left index finger in front of my nose, and performed the cover test right there. When I covered one of his eyes, the other eye jumped outward. I went back and forth between both eyes several times. The magnitude of jumping was more on the right eye than on the left eye.

"Do you know how to count fingers?" I asked Sean. He nodded and demonstrated it to me.

I quickly moved the smiley face from my index finger to my nose; the sticker remained there barely long enough for me to do the finger-counting confrontation visual field test on him. I wanted to confirm that his visual field was full, and it was.

"Yeah, Sean's eyes are not aligned. He needs a comprehensive eye exam soon," I urged the mother. She asked me where I practiced. Coincidently, they lived about ten miles away from our office. What a small world!

The following week, Sean and both his parents showed up in our office. Sean received a comprehensive eye exam with cycloplegic drops, used to relax his focusing system temporarily to determine his eye condition. His right eye had about 40 prism diopters esotropia, a condition in which the eye turns inward due to the eye muscles' imbalance. His left eye had 20 prism diopters esotropia. The deviation was about the same both distant and near. Both eyes had 2 diopters of hyperopia or farsightedness. The best correctable vision was worse in the right eye due to the presence of strabismus amblyopia. He had no depth perception (3-D perception) based on the random dot stereopsis test. Stereopsis or stereovision is also called depth perception.

YOUR PRECIOUS SIGHT

Stereovision is how each eye may see an object from a different angle but combines these angles in the brain to give us a 3-D image. When one's eyes are not working as a team, there is no 3-D perception.

His father hunched his shoulders; his mother sank back into the armchair. Neither parent could conceal their profound worries about their son's eyes affecting his learning and dimming his bright future. I could relate to that well.

I discussed the treatment options with the parents, which included eye surgery and combinations of prescription lenses, eye patching, and visual training (vision therapy). Both parents were apprehensive about the surgery.

To ensure that Sean's vision would not hinder his close-up work and reading, he was given a pair of bifocals with base-out prisms. I have to admit that there was some guessing involved in the prescription. I also referred him to my colleague, who specialized in pediatric vision and visual training. In vision therapy, he would learn how to use the two eyes together in hopes of improving his eyes' alignment and binocular vision, in which both eyes work as a team to see the same visual target at the same time, equally and accurately.

When Sean was six years old, his parents warmed up to the idea of surgery, so I referred him to a strabismus surgeon. He received the surgery on both eyes to adjust the strength of his ocular muscles and straighten his eyes' alignment.

Sean wore single vision lenses with full hyperopic correction afterward. He continued visual training and patching his left eye to enhance his binocular vision, with full support from both parents. He could stop eye patching once the best correctable vision on both eyes was the same.

The summer after fourth grade, Sean's father's engineering firm transferred him to Houston, Texas. His whole family decided to relocate.

At Sean's last eye exam, the stereovision test showed that he had some depth perception, though not perfect; however, it was better than none at all. I encouraged him to keep up the visual training so he could enjoy 3-D movies as his friends did. For many people, crossed eyes are a cosmetic issue. However, it is as relevant visually as cosmetically.

"He's an honor student, number one in his entire fourth grade," his father proudly told me as he shook my hand zealously before departing.

I cannot wait to hear that the patient I met in Las Vegas got accepted to MIT or one of the Ivy League schools!

~ * ~

I like to share with you a statement from the American Association for Pediatric Ophthalmology and Strabismus:

"**Amblyopia** was associated with slower reading speed in school-age children. Treatment for monocular amblyopia visual acuity impairment could improve reading speed and efficiency."

Children with amblyopia make more corrective eye movements while reading and read slower than normally sighted children. The American Optometric Association recommends that all children have their first eye exam at six months of age, another exam at age three, and a third exam prior to entering school to ensure vision is developing normally in both eyes and there is no risk of amblyopia.

The treatments of amblyopia involve providing full correction to both eyes, strabismus surgery to align the eyes if necessary, eye patching, and vision therapy. The ultimate goal is to have both eyes work together uniformly as a team so that the brain can receive clear and simultaneous stimulation from each eye. Amblyopia will not diminish by itself or be outgrown.

For more information, please check out the References section at the back, under Chapter 1.

YOUR PRECIOUS SIGHT

Chapter Key Points:

- The purpose of patching the good eye is to force the weak eye to work in hopes of improving its best correctable vision.
- If the amblyopia is caused by significant reflective error, like nearsightedness, farsightedness, or astigmatism, the patient needs to wear the corrective eyewear—glasses or contact lenses—full time.
- For strabismus patients, the goal of visual training is to improve the eyes' alignment and binocular vision so that both eyes work as a team, seeing the same visual target at the same time equally and accurately.
- Every child should have at least one comprehensive eye exam by age three, before entering preschool.
- According to research, amblyopia is associated with slower reading speed and learning efficiency.
- Strabismus, or lazy eye, cannot be outgrown, nor will it improve by itself.

Chapter 2

"My child cannot differentiate colors."

The Stories of Color Deficiency

"Most of us share a common color vision sensory experience. Some people, however, have a color vision deficiency, which means their perception of colors is different from what most of us see. The most severe forms of these deficiencies are referred to as color blindness. People with color blindness aren't aware of differences among colors that are obvious to the rest of us. People who don't have the more severe types of color blindness may not even be aware of their condition unless they're tested in a clinic or laboratory."

~NIH

WHEN I ENTERED the exam room, Kenny

was sitting on his mother's lap while she read a picture book to him. He looked up at me and gave me a big-boy "hi."

My technician had given me a heads-up about the age of this kid, so I had taken off my white jacket. It always works better with little kids to eliminate the possible association of a white coat with painful shots.

"Hi! What a big boy! How old are you, sweetheart?" Kids at this age still possess the sweet innocence and purity that make you want to pull them in and hug them tight.

He popped up four fingers.

Before I asked any questions, his mother eagerly told me her concerns. "Kenny has no difficulties learning numbers or letters. He's one of the fast learners in that area in his preschool. But he is struggling with his colors. We have taught him the colors for a couple of months, but he still picks up the wrong colors of crayons."

I looked at the pretest results and noticed that he missed all fifteen plates of the Ishihara color test. Since his mother had mentioned that he knew numbers, I used a piece of paper and a black marker to play the number game with him. Indeed, he knew all the numbers I asked.

He even named the two-digit numbers correctly.

"Is there any family history of color deficiency? It was called color blindness in the past," I said.

"I have no idea. We adopted him when he was an infant," his mother said. "He is our only child. We love him very much."

"You are a loving mother. I can tell that easily. Kenny is lucky to have you."

I did all the comprehensive eye exams with him. With some coaxing, little Kenny even let me put the eye drops in to dilate his eyes. With the picture eye chart, the best he could see was 20/40 with mild farsightedness.

The diagnosis was that he had some form of color deficiency. I did not prescribe him eyewear, because it's not an uncommon issue for kids at that age with slight farsightedness. However, it was difficult to pinpoint the severity or the exact form of color deficiency. I communicated the results to his mother.

"Can it be cured?" His mother appeared apprehensive and grave.

I explained to her that Kenny's color deficiency

is a genetic condition and there's no cure. A comprehensive color disk test like the 100 Hue Test, arranging colored disks to a smooth gradient, would provide a more precise diagnosis of Kenny's color deficiencies. However, it's a lengthy and elaborate test for someone his age; it would not provide much meaningful information at this point in his development.

I encouraged his mother to continue reading books, drawing, and practicing tracing lines on paper with him to develop his hand-eye coordination. A vision report was prepared for the mother to inform the schoolteacher.

Kenny's mother brought him back for follow-up yearly. He gradually shifted from mild farsightedness to nearsightedness. In fourth grade, he received a pair of glasses. His best correctable vision maintained at 20/40. While a person with 20/20 vision can see an object at twenty feet, Kenny had to move up to ten feet to see it. He was also diagnosed with severe blue-yellow and moderate red-green color deficiency with a hue-arranging test at that time.

Despite his vision problem, Kenny's grades stayed above the average level, and he was well-liked in school by his teachers and friends, as his mother reported.

~ * ~

"Red-green color vision defects are the most common form of color vision deficiency. This condition affects males much more often than females. Red-green color vision defects and blue cone monochromacy are inherited in an X-linked recessive pattern. The OPN1LW and OPN1MW genes are located on the X chromosome, which is one of the two sex chromosomes. In males (who have only one X chromosome), one genetic change in each cell is sufficient to cause the condition. Males are affected by X-linked recessive disorders much more frequently than females because in females (who have two X chromosomes), a genetic change would have to occur on both copies of the chromosome to cause the disorder. A characteristic of X-linked inheritance is that fathers cannot pass X-linked traits to their sons."

~NIH

JOSE WAS A 20-year-old, well-built young

man. His red-green color deficiency was diagnosed when he was seven years old. However, being a police officer had always been his dream, even though he was aware of the restriction on the police academy application regarding the color vision requirement. On the LAPD (Los Angeles Police Department) application, it stated that "candidates must be able to accurately and quickly name colors."

The retina, located at the back of the eye's interior, contains light-and-color wavelength-sensitive cells referred to as rods and cones, which transmit relevant information to the brain to process the color perception.

There are special glasses and contact lenses on the market to enhance the color perception of color-deficient patients with various levels of success. How much a person can benefit from this kind of lens depends on the severity and the type of abnormality in retina photopigments, aka rods and cones.

Jose understood the situation; nevertheless, he was motivated to give it a shot, even if there was no guarantee. A deep-red x-chrome soft contact lens was fitted on his nondominant eye as recommended by the manufacturer who designed this lens. It helped him differentiate colors better but not perfectly. He did not pass the qualifying vision test for the police academy, which was a disappointment. He shifted his career goals toward becoming a radiology technician.

It is estimated that eight percent of men and 0.5 percent of women were born with color deficiency.

It's strongly recommended that every child has a comprehensive eye exam before entering preschool, including a color test. Early diagnosis of color deficiency can help a child receive support and understanding from family and teachers. Later on, children can use this information to obtain the proper career guidance with the help of occupational consultants.

Although this chapter focuses on genetic color deficiency, there are certain medications and illnesses that can cause adult-acquired color vision deficiency.

For more information, please check out the References section at the back, under Chapter 2.

YOUR PRECIOUS SIGHT

Chapter Key Points:

- Red-green color vision defects are the most common form of color vision deficiency.
- Another form of color deficiency is blue-yellow. This is a rarer and more severe form of color vision loss than red-green, because people with blue-yellow deficiency frequently have red-green blindness too.
- Color deficiency is most often a genetic condition caused by a common X-linked recessive gene.
- It is estimated that eight percent of men and 0.5 percent of women were born with color deficiency.
- Early diagnosis of color deficiency can help a child receive support and understanding from family and teachers and obtain proper career guidance when the time comes to do so.
- Certain diseases or injury can be damaging to the optic nerve or retina and may alter a person's color perception and recognition.
- Medications like those used to treat heart problems, high blood pressure, infections, nervous disorders, autoimmune diseases,

and psychological problems can affect color vision.

Chapter 3

"I want to wear contact lenses, but my mother said no."

When is the Right Age to Introduce Contact Lenses to Youngsters?

"The U.S. Food and Drug Administration regulates contact lenses and certain contact lens care products as medical devices. Best strategies for reducing your risk of infection involve proper hygiene; following recommended wearing schedules; using proper lens care practices for cleaning, disinfecting and storing your lenses (which includes reading and following all product labeling instructions); and having routine eye exams."

~US Food and Drug Administration (FDA)

I COMMUNICATED THE findings to the

patient, Cynthia, and her mother after completing the eye exam. I turned toward Cynthia, a 10-year-old girl, giving her a quick reminder about taking care of glasses. She stared at me, oblivious, as if all I'd said was, "Blah, blah, blah."

Cynthia turned to her mother, who was seated on the armchair in the corner, and said in a demanding voice, "I want contact lenses!"

"You are not ready yet." Her mother was calm, as she had been waiting for this moment to say those words.

"What do you mean? Lots of my friends at school are wearing contact lenses!"

"Let's wait for a couple more years when you are more responsible."

"I want them *now*!"

Observing the dynamics between mother and daughter, I recalled my own kids at that age.

"Why do you want to wear contact lenses?" I asked Cynthia. She had 2 diopters of nearsightedness and 1 diopter of astigmatism. Nowadays, there are many contact lens options to fit her in terms of types and modalities. However, my concern was not with finding the right

YOUR PRECIOUS SIGHT

brand for her prescription; it was her motivation for wearing contact lenses that I found disconcerting.

"I want to change my eye color. My friend has blue contact lenses," she replied.

"I think you should listen to your mom. Contact lenses rest right on your corneas, the front part of your eyes. A contact lens is a medical device. It's not like a pair of shoes that you can slip on and go. It requires a lot of diligent care, or you can go blind from cornea infection." Cynthia pursed her lips while she listened to what I was saying.

"I know how to take care of contact lenses. I've seen my friend doing it," Cynthia muttered.

"What is the right age for kids to start wearing contact lenses?" her mother queried.

"Age is not the first consideration," I told her. "It's all about whether the person is mature enough to accept the responsibility of caring for contact lenses. A contact lens is a medical device; you can't mess around with it."

I decided to share with them the most unpleasant case I had experienced during my early optometric career. The patient, a man in his thirties who was an account executive for a startup company, traveled internationally. For his convenience and practical needs, I fitted him with one-day disposable lenses. He signed off on all the forms, stating that he fully understood that the lenses were not for overnight wear. He was instructed to remove the lenses and discard them every night.

More than one year passed, one day he came in with swollen, painful, red eyes. The right eye was more so than the left. He was *still* wearing his contact lenses! I could see an opaque diffuse area in the center of his right eye even without the microscope. It must have been greater than three millimeters!

Since my office did not have the media to perform the microbial culture, I removed his contact lenses and put them into a contact lens container with sterilized saline solution for the lab to do the culture. His contact lenses were discolored and *filthy*!

He told me that he had been out of the States, and the trip had dragged on much longer than originally planned. He had run out of contact lenses, so the same pair had been in his eyes for three months without removal.

YOUR PRECIOUS SIGHT

The fluorescein stain indicated that he had a severe case of infectious keratitis (corneal ulcers) in both eyes, more threatening in the right eye. A great percentage of corneal ulcers are caused by the malicious bug called Pseudomonas, which can penetrate the cornea in just a few hours. I drowned his eyes with an antibiotic solution and then referred him to the general ophthalmologist across the street immediately.

For the next two years, the ophthalmologist kept me updated on the development of this patient. To make a long story short, even after the patient's corneal ulcers were treated and healed, the large, dense scars on his eyes had substantially distorted his corneas, particularly on the right eye, which impeded his daily function. The ophthalmologist referred him to a corneal specialist to have a corneal transplant on the right eye. The first transplant failed, and he needed another.

Even though I bore no liability for his suffering and vision loss, knowing the ordeal this patient had to endure disturbed me.

After listening to my story, Cynthia hung her head. Her mother gently told her, "How about if you bring up your math grade from C to B and get no tardy reports from the school in this school year, then you'll get contact lenses at your next yearly eye exam?"

"Okay," Cynthia responded reluctantly.

It's not an overstatement that contact lenses can cause blindness if a patient does not diligently follow guidelines and protocols.

Furthermore, *all* contact lens wearers should possess a pair of updated glasses as a backup, especially during traveling or when battling a cold or flu. Your eyes do need a break every so often. After all, contact lenses are, in reality, *foreign bodies* to our eyeballs.

~ * ~

"They are not cosmetics or over-the-counter merchandise. They are medical devices regulated by the U.S. Food and Drug Administration. Places that advertise them as cosmetics or sell them over-the-counter, without a prescription, are breaking the law."

~FDA

YOUR PRECIOUS SIGHT

GISELE, AN 18-YEAR-OLD freshman at the local community college, came in for an emergency red-eye exam. My assistant took her to the exam room directly without pretesting, the procedure we abide by for most of the red-eye/pink-eye patients.

After reviewing her case history, I removed her green contact lenses. Her beautiful, dark-brown eyes revealed sick cornea—diffused punctate staining with marginal infiltrates and bloodshot conjunctiva (the white part of the eye), which is usually an indication of imminent cornea infection if it had not already happened.

"Where did you get your contact lenses?" I questioned her. I could tell what type of contact lenses she wore just by looking at them; nevertheless, I wanted to know who dispensed the lenses so I could ask for her previous eye care information.

"I got them from somewhere." She averted her eyes.

"Do you have the doctor's name? My front office can call to get your contact lens information." Truthfully, I could go through the exam without any previous information. It would be helpful but not detrimental without it.

However, her dubious look drove me to press her further.

"I got them from the swap meet," she finally admitted.

"Do you go to the swap meet for your painful red eyes?" The exasperation surged up in me.

"No."

"So, why did you get them there if the place could not take care of you?" I said, my tone harsh.

I did take care of her painful red eyes with a run of antibiotic-steroid-combination eye drops. She also got an earful from me.

It concerns me more than irritates me when I learn a patient has obtained contact lenses from places like swap meets, gas stations, beauty salons, or sidewalk vendors. Those people who dispense contact lenses without license and training are criminals; they should go to jail!

The public needs to be educated on the fact that a contact lens is a medical device, a foreign body to our eye. The eyes need to be thoroughly examined, and the curvature of the corneas needs to be measured so the doctor can determine the most suitable lenses for particular eyes. Patients need to be trained on how to handle and care for the lenses. Also, regular follow-ups are required to ensure the health of the eyes is not affected by contact lens wearing.

Contact lenses, if not properly worn or taken care of, can cause blindness!

For more information about *Healthy Contact Lens Wear & Care,* please check out the References section at the back under Chapter 3.

IN OUR OFFICE, we have a handout for contact lens wearers who use cosmetics. I acquired this information, titled "Contact Lenses and Cosmetics," from the American Optometric Association website.

You can wear contacts and cosmetics safely and comfortably together by following these helpful tips:

- Put on soft contact lenses before applying makeup.
- Put on rigid gas-permeable (RGP) lenses after applying makeup.

- Avoid lash-extending mascara, which has fibers that can irritate the eyes. Also, avoid waterproof mascara, which cannot be easily removed with water and may stain soft contact lenses. Replace mascara at least every three months.
- Avoid applying eyeliner along the watermark of the eyelid.
- Remove lenses before removing makeup.
- Choose an oil-free moisturizer.
- Don't use hand creams or lotions before handling contacts. They can leave a film on your lenses.
- Use hairspray before putting on your contacts. If you use hairspray while you are wearing your contacts, close your eyes during spraying and for a few seconds after.
- Blink your eyes frequently while using a hair dryer to keep your eyes from getting too dry.
- Keep false eyelash cement, nail polish and remover, perfume, and cologne away from lenses. They can damage the plastic.
- Choose water-based, hypoallergenic liquid foundations. Cream makeup may leave a film on your lenses.

YOUR PRECIOUS SIGHT

Chapter Key Points:

- Contact lenses and certain contact lens care products are regulated by the U.S. Food and Drug Administration as *medical devices*.
- A great percentage of corneal ulcers are caused by the malicious bug called Pseudomonas. It can penetrate the cornea in just a few hours, develop a permanent scar, and lead to vision loss.
- *ALL* contact lens wearers should possess a pair of glasses with updated prescription as a backup, especially during traveling or having a cold or flu.
- Remove contact lenses *immediately* if eye irritation occurs.
- Places that advertise colored contact lenses as cosmetics or sell them over the counter without an updated contact lens prescription from a licensed eyecare professional are doing so illegally.
- Best approaches for reducing your risk of infection include proper hygiene, such as washing hands thoroughly before handling contact lenses and touching eyes; following recommended wearing schedules and regimen; disposing of lenses as prescribed; using

proper lens care systems for cleaning and disinfecting; storing lenses in fresh solution and a clean case; reading and following all product labeling instructions; and having routine eye exams.
- Dispose of eye makeup every three months.

Chapter 4

"We had so much fun at the makeover party!"

The Stories of Conjunctivitis (Red Eye/Pink Eye)

---

*"**Pink eye**, also known as **conjunctivitis**, involves inflammation of the conjunctiva, the thin, clear tissue that lines the inside of the eyelid and covers the white part of the eye, or sclera. The inflammation makes blood vessels more visible, giving the eye a pink or reddish appearance. The affected eye(s) may be painful, itchy or have a burning sensation. The eyes can also tear or have a discharge that forms a crust during sleep, causing the eyes to be 'stuck shut' in the morning."*

~NEI

ON A TYPICAL Monday morning, patients

lined up outside the front door before the office opened at 9 a. m. Things tend to happen during the weekend: glasses fly off on the Batman ride at Six Flags Magic Mountain, dogs chew on glasses, and things get into the eyes.

I waited in my exam room in jump-right-into-action mode. My assistant guided the first walk-in patient, Sarah, a 16-year-old girl, and her grandmother into the room.

"Her mother is at work, so I brought her in. She woke up with red eyes," the grandmother said.

"What happened when you first woke up this morning?" I asked Sarah.

"My lids were kind of glued together. I had to wash my face to get them open. They're sore and red."

No kidding. Her eyes were cherry-red with some mucus accumulating at the inner corners or nasal canthus.

Her cornea and the anterior chamber, the front segment of eyes, were normal through the slip lamp (microscope) examination.

My diagnosis was bacterial conjunctivitis, a

YOUR PRECIOUS SIGHT

bacterial infection. I wrote her a prescription for an antibiotic ophthalmic solution and instructed her to return right away if the condition got worse.

Right after lunch, my assistant handed me two charts. "Twins. Both are walk-ins with red eyes. Mother is with them."

I looked at the names and dates of birth and stepped into the exam room.

"Happy belated birthday!" I said to them. "You both just had your big day."

The girls gave me toothy smiles. *They were identical!*

"So, who is Kelly? Who is Kera?"

They identified themselves simultaneously. I quickly jotted down the color of their dental braces on their charts—Kelly's were blue; Kera's were pink—and noticed they both had red, mucus-filled eyes like Sarah's.

"Their friend Sarah came in this morning for pink eye, and you gave her eye drops. It seems like Kelly and Kera have the same thing," their mother explained.

The one with pink braces added, "She texted me about it."

I started my case history. "Did you guys do anything together this weekend?"

"We reserved a room at the Holiday Inn. They invited a few friends to have a makeover and sleepover party for their sixteenth birthdays," the mother said.

"Everyone brought their makeup kits. We shared…"

"Brenda had some cool contact lenses. We all tried them on," Kelly cut in before Kera completed her sentence.

"What you mean by 'cool' contact lenses?" I inquired.

"There was one pair like cat eyes," Kelly recounted, "and one like vampire's eyes and one had a star on it."

I was alarmed. "Do you know where she got those contact lenses?"

"She said she got them in Mexico City."

I'd heard enough and needed to get going. Like Sarah, they both had bacterial conjunctivitis.

"You guys not only shared your makeup and contact lenses, but you shared the bugs as

YOUR PRECIOUS SIGHT

well," I told them.

"Do you share your undies?" Sometimes I asked teenagers over-the-top, provocative questions to get their minds operating.

"Yuck! That's gross!" They squealed in unison.

"What made you think your eyes were less important?" I said. Their mother gave me a nod.

Besides prescribing antibiotic eye drops, I instructed them to throw all the used makeup away and to never, ever, share makeup. I also provided information regarding basic ocular hygiene.

I knew another patient was waiting in the next exam room, so I ended with a quick lecture about the importance of treating contact lenses as a medical device.

*"**Viral conjunctivitis** is often diagnosed based on a person's history and symptoms. It tends to occur in both eyes and often accompanies a common cold or respiratory tract*

infection. Laboratory tests usually are not needed to diagnose viral conjunctivitis; however, testing may be done if a more severe form of viral conjunctivitis is suspected. More severe causes include herpes simplex virus (which usually involves blisters on the skin), varicella-zoster virus (chickenpox and shingles), rubella or rubeola (measles). This testing is performed using a sample of the discharge from an infected eye."

~NEI

TWO OF MY assistants called in sick; something was going around. It's stressful when the office is short-staffed. I took 1,000 mg of vitamin C to boost up my immunity.

Rodney cuddled with his mother in the armchair and coughed his head off when I walked into the room. He was five years old and going to kindergarten.

"He had a cold for two days, and his pediatrician gave him cold syrup. There's no more fever, but I noticed his eyes turned really red and watery today." Rodney was whining between coughs while his mother talked to me.

Based on what I heard and observed, I decided

not to put him behind the slit lamp. I used a penlight to check his pupillary reaction and ocular motility. Everything appeared normal except for the watery, red eyes.

The diagnosis was that Rodney had viral conjunctivitis.

I told his mother that if it got worse in the next three to four days, she should bring him back. Otherwise, it should run its course and clear up within the next week or two. Most likely, the tearing and crusty eyes would resolve within three to seven days. He should stay home during this time. I explained that Rodney and the other family members needed to wash their hands frequently and avoid touching their eyes. Everyone should have individual hand and wash towels to limit the contamination.

The mother nodded while suppressing a yawn.

I repeated the line, "Viral conjunctivitis is very contagious!" several times to ensure the mother got the message.

Once the patient left, the exam room—especially the armchair area—was sprayed with a disinfectant solution. Let me reiterate that most viral eye infections are self-limiting, like flu; they eventually run their course without intervention. However, they can be extremely contagious. They can spread from one eye to the other eye. They can also spread to other family members and schoolmates and lead to outbreaks if precautions, like washing hands and not sharing towels, are not implemented.

I also want to mention that some sexually transmitted diseases (STDs) can occur in the eyes and can mimic less-serious eye conditions such as the pink eye. For example, herpes, syphilis, gonorrhea, chlamydia, venereal warts, HIV/AIDS, and pubic lice can all cause eye infection and inflammation. Some of the STD eye diseases are extremely dangerous. They require prompt care and aggressive treatment to avoid adversely affecting vision permanently. Blindness caused by STD eye infection is not uncommon.

The bottom line is, not all pink eye has the same etiology. You should have a thorough eye exam when in doubt.

For more information, please check out the References section at the back, under Chapter 4.

Chapter Key Points:

- Throw away your eye makeup and purchase a fresh supply every three months. Bacteria can grow rapidly, especially on liquid eye makeup.
- Never, ever, share contact lenses, makeup, or applicators with anyone.
- Remove all eye makeup at night before sleeping.
- If you develop an eye infection, throw away your contact lenses and *all* eye makeup immediately to avoid reinfection.
- You can get red eye/pink eye from various etiologies: infections (bacteria, fungi, viruses, or parasite), allergies, or chemical toxic reaction.
- Viruses cause up to eighty percent of conjunctivitis. Infectious pink eye is prevalent among schoolchildren and is very contagious.
- The best strategies for limiting the spread of viral conjunctivitis are washing hands frequently, and no hand/facial towel sharing.
- Not all red eye/pink eye has the same etiology. When sexually transmitted diseases

(STDs) affect the eyes, they become dangerously serious. Historically, red eye induced by sexually transmitted eye infections has been one of the leading causes of blindness worldwide.

Chapter 5

"Can I tie his hands to stop him from rubbing his eyes?"

The Stories of Eye Allergies

*"**Eye allergies**, also called **allergic conjunctivitis**, are a common eye condition. The tissue that lines the inside of the eyelid and outside of the eyeball is called the conjunctiva. This tissue keeps your eyelid and eyeball moist. Allergic conjunctivitis occurs when this tissue becomes inflamed. With eye allergies, you usually see redness and itching in both eyes, instead of in just one eye.*

~Asthma and Allergy Foundation of America

THE HALLMARK OF ocular allergy is itchiness and clear, watery discharge. The symptoms can range from mild to severe. One of the most severe cases I have encountered was when I was in my fourth year of optometry school, interning at Omni Eye Clinic in Phoenix, Arizona.

A 9-year-old boy, Ramón Lopez, sat in the reception area. His eyes hid behind oversized sunglasses he'd apparently borrowed from an adult. He was sniffing and wiping his nose with a handful of used tissues. I introduced myself but omitted the step of shaking hands with him, which I usually do while offering a friendly greeting to break the ice.

He is sick. And, probably contagious. I will dismiss him in no time. I thought as I looked at him. While I walked him to the exam room, he continued to cough and sniffle.

He climbed up on the exam chair and took off the sunglasses. I let him hand them directly to the accompanying adult, his older sister.

"His eyes are very red. How long has this been going on?" I asked the sister without taking my eyes off his face. I noticed the discharge was clear.

"He rubbed his eyes a lot. I told him not to do it, but he didn't listen." His older sister sounded frustrated.

YOUR PRECIOUS SIGHT

"My eyes are itchy, and they hurt," Ramón protested.

When I heard the word "itchy," I let down my guard. I made a differential diagnosis: he had an allergy, not a cold. An allergy is an immunological issue and is *not* contagious. Through the case history, I learned that he had previously visited a primary care physician and received oral medication for allergies; however, it did not seem to help his itchy, red eyes.

It stunned me when I everted his upper lids. There were pebble-like bumps packed tightly on the upper tarsal conjunctiva. His cornea was covered with punctate stainings. It was no wonder that he was light-sensitive and miserable.

My staff doctor then guided me through the diagnosis and treatment plan. Vernal keratoconjunctivitis is also known as cobblestone conjunctivitis. It's an inflammatory disease in response to environmental allergens like pollen, dust mites, and animal dander. In many cases, it's season-related. The treatment is usually a combination of long-term topical mast cell stabilizers and antihistamines, with short-term use of topical corticosteroids in addition to the removal of the allergens.

"Use a cold compress if your eyes get itchy," I told the boy. I explained to Ramón and his sister how to do a cold compress with a clean, wet towel placed in the refrigerator for ten minutes before rolling it up and placing it on the eyes.

"He rubs his eyes so hard. My mother is afraid that he's going blind." His sister's concern was palpable.

"When you rub your eyes, you promote the release of histamine and make your eyes itchier." I communicated with Ramón, as he was a big boy.

"Maybe we should tie his hands with a rope if he rubs his eyes," the sister said, narrowing her eyes as she glared at Ramón.

"I'm not sure you should go that far," I said.

With the treatment, his symptoms subsided in one week. Nevertheless, the angry look of the upper tarsal conjunctiva took much longer to heal. The topical corticosteroids were tapered off after one week to avoid the side effect of increasing the intraocular pressure, which may lead to glaucoma.

~ * ~

YOUR PRECIOUS SIGHT

*"**Blepharitis** is an inflammation of the eyelids in which they become red, irritated and itchy, and dandruff-like scales form on the eyelashes. It is a common eye disorder caused by either bacteria or a skin condition, such as dandruff of the scalp or rosacea. It affects people of all ages."*

~AOA

NICOLA, A LOCAL college senior, accompanied by her boyfriend, walked into the office as it opened one morning.

Her eyelids were swollen shut. I did not like the way it looked, and I felt my stomach lurch.

She'd been in the office ten days before, complaining of crusty scales, lids stuck together in the morning, and red eyes. The diagnosis was blepharitis and a mild bacterial infection. I prescribed her Bacitracin ophthalmic ointment 500unit/gram three times a day for a week. The reason for ointment versus the solution was its longer retention time in the eye. I did mention to her about the blurred vision caused by the ointment and advised her not to drive while using it. However, I could not recall whether I had warned her of the side effects of Bacitracin. Reviewing her chart, I did not find that I had done so.

Now, my gut twisted and tightened into knots. Nausea billowed within me. I drew in a deep breath, slowly and silently exhaled.

It was quite possible that she'd suffered an allergic reaction to the sulfa component of the medication. I had her discontinue the ointment immediately, which she should have done three days before.

Since she did not display a life-threatening type of allergic reaction, like anaphylaxis, I did not send her to the emergency room. However, I warned her about the signs and symptoms of anaphylaxis and Stevens-Johnson syndrome. This time I made sure to write it down on the chart that I'd done so.

I washed her eyes thoroughly with sterilized saline and non-preservative artificial tears and prescribed her over-the-counter antihistamines. When she returned to the office for a follow-up two days later, the condition had improved dramatically. I let out a sigh of relief.

Sulfa is not the only scoundrel in ophthalmic products causing an allergic or toxic reaction. Some agents, like thimerosal, used as a preservative in contact lens solutions, can cause follicular conjunctivitis, giant papillary conjunctivitis, or contact dermatitis.

In recent years, the eye care industry has tested and experimented with various kinds of preservatives and claimed the incidents of adverse reaction have diminished from two decades ago. Clinically, I have witnessed fewer cases of red or itchy eyes related to contact lens solution use. However, the one-day disposable contacts lenses modality and hydrogen peroxide care system are my preferred alternatives for contact lens wearers. Also, I strongly recommend preservative-free, single-dose artificial tears for dry eye patients.

Chapter Key Points:

- The primary signs of ocular allergy are red, itchy eyes and clear, watery discharge.
- The most common allergens that cause eye allergies are pollen, mold, dust, and animal dander.
- Chemicals in certain cosmetics and preservatives in some eye drops/contact lens cleaning solutions can cause eye allergies as well.
- Besides the avoidance of allergens, one of the best ways to reduce itchiness is by applying a cold compress.
- Rubbing eyes provokes the release of histamine and promote the itchiness; moreover, you may scratch your cornea. Do not rub your eyes!
- The incidence of allergic reaction to a certain component in ophthalmic medication or eye care solution is low. However, if you experience any unusual reaction, like itchiness, eyelid swelling or crusting, tearing, or sensitivity to light, you should contact your doctor immediately.

Chapter 6

"She smashed the car!"

The Stories of Retinitis Pigmentosa

"Retinitis pigmentosa (RP) is a group of rare, genetic disorders that involve a breakdown and loss of cells in the retina. Common symptoms include difficulty seeing at night and a loss of side (peripheral) vision. The retina is the light-sensitive tissue at the back of the eye that contains photoreceptors and other cell types."

~NIH

"THE LAST PATIENT is ready for you," my technician informed me when I walked toward the front office with the contact lenses follow-up patient.

The office had two examination rooms. To

make the flow run efficiently, I rotated between them. I was surprised to see both Mr. and Mrs. Smithson in the room with their daughter, Kailyn. Mrs. Smithson was the one who usually brought her two boys to have eye exams. I hadn't seen Kailyn for a few years. She was the only one in the family who had perfect vision, unlike her two older brothers who had worn glasses since elementary school. They used to tease her that she was adopted.

"How's life treating you?" I asked. I like to learn more about each patient as a person instead of just focusing on their eyes.

Kailyn, who just had her sixteenth birthday, did not look up; she was looking at her iPhone, probably glued to one of the social media sites. Mrs. Smithson elbowed her husband, who exhaled long and loud before speaking.

"She smashed the car into the side of the garage the other night," he stated.

"Wow. How did that happen?" I turned to look at Kailyn and asked.

"Someone parked the car too close to the side. It wasn't my fault." Kailyn looked up briefly; her eyes filled with contempt. Before waiting for my next question, her father spoke up.

YOUR PRECIOUS SIGHT

"She said she had passed driver's education in school and had the provisional permit. She needed some practice on the road. My wife thought I was the perfect candidate to help her. I was forced into that job. God knows why. I did a couple of times with her on the weekend, during the daytime, and she did alright. I was tired when I got home the other night. Both Kailyn and my wife bugged me to practice with her. She backed up the car too fast. Before I knew it, the car smashed into the side of the garage door. The rear light on the passenger side broke in pieces. She insisted that she didn't see it."

"She tripped over the dog in the hallway the other night," Mrs. Smithson said. "She complained and insisted that I'd made it too dark in there. It was the same light bulb that had been there for months."

One good thing about being the last patient was that I didn't have the pressure of knowing that another patient was waiting for me in the next room. Therefore, I let the parents express their concerns. In the meantime, I paid attention to Kailyn's reactions. I knew she feigned ignorance; however, her mind was engaged in the conversation. When smashing the car and tripping over the dog were mentioned, she rolled her eyes.

After learning enough of the case, I jumped right into the exam. The results confirmed my suspicion. Kailyn had a constricted visual field. The digital retinal photo through her dilated eyes showed the pigment deposit in the typical bone-spicule formation at mid-fundus.

I communicated the diagnosis with her parents and Kailyn: she had a genetic condition called Retinitis Pigmentosa (RP).

"Is she going blind?" her father asked.

"RP is a progressive disease, but it's hard to predict the rate of visual loss. Most patients become legally blind by the age of forty." I tried to choose my words with discretion and deliver the facts at the same time. The devastation radiating from the parents disheartened me. I recalled the day when I was in their position, when the audiologist told me that my son was profoundly deaf and would never call me "mother" in words.

Since I was confident in my diagnosis, and to save them from another doctor visit, I did not refer them for a second opinion. Instead, I referred them to the Center for the Partially Sighted in Los Angeles. It may seem a bit too

YOUR PRECIOUS SIGHT

abrupt and harsh; however, I think it's beneficial for the patient and family to learn about prospects and prepare for the process of vision decline at this stage.

The Center for the Partially Sighted is a nonprofit organization run by optometrists specialized in low vision practice. At some centers, there are social workers, support groups, and psychologists to provide support to the patient and family. The patients will learn to use some low-vision aids while they still have a decent vision and can gradually adjust their lifestyles.

While I walked them to the front office, I heard Kailyn whisper to her mother, "I just want to get my driver's license. All of my friends have driver's licenses already." She was in the denial phase; I could understand that.

I looked at the parents. Mr. Smithson appeared impassive with a stoic front, and Mrs. Smithson was composed. I'd known the mother for a few years and considered her a friend. I turned and gave her a tight hug; she reciprocated. When I pull away, I saw the glistening of tears at the corners of her eyes. I knew she would go home and cry. That's what I did years ago.

DR. EICHIN CHANG-LIM

~ * ~

*"**Usher syndrome** is the most common condition that affects both hearing and vision; sometimes it also affects balance. The major symptoms of Usher syndrome are deafness or hearing loss and an eye disease called retinitis pigmentosa (RP)."*

~NIH

JASON GRADUATED FROM high school not long ago. He was born severely hearing impaired and communicated with sign language. He came in by himself on that day. His mother used to accompany him and interpret for him when needed. Since my son is an oral-deaf with a cochlear implant, my sign language was limited, so I communicated with Jason by paper and pen.

He complained that his glasses were getting "weak" and that he could not see well at night.

He had passed the vision test and obtained his driver's license a year ago. I performed a comprehensive exam. His best correctible vision had worsened from 20/20 a couple of years ago to 20/30. His retina exhibited pigment deposits, like the patient I mentioned previously.

I displayed his digital fundus photos on the monitor, along with his previous ones, and showed them to him. The changes were unmistakable. He had a genetic condition called Usher syndrome.

The primary symptoms of Usher syndrome are hearing loss and retinitis pigmentosa. It is a disorder that affects both hearing and vision.

I encountered two dilemmas and contemplated my strategies while walking him from the camera room to the exam room. First, he was over eighteen years old. To comply with HIPAA privacy rules, I could not communicate the findings with his mother, even though a sense of urgency compelled me to do so. Secondly, he possessed a valid driver's license. I wondered if I had the right or will to revoke it.

Again, I communicated with him in the exam room using a pen and paper. He promised me that he would tell his mother as soon as he got home. While I was uncertain I was doing the right thing, the guidelines I gave him regarding his driving were:

- Stop driving before sunset.
- No driving on rainy or overcast days.

- No freeway driving.
- Do not drive over the speed limit.
- Avoid changing lanes. Be sure turn your head and look over your shoulder if changing lanes is needed.

He was aware of the dangers of driving and the possibility of losing his driver's license. He told me he took buses sometimes; I applauded him for doing so.

I referred him to the St. Mary Low Vision Center in Long Beach, which was closer and more convenient for him. At the same time, I gave him the name and contact information of the local Department of Rehabilitation. A counselor there, who was a sign-deaf, had provided support and guidance to my son since he was in high school. The Department of Rehab would do a battery of tests and a questionnaire to determine the appropriate vocational training and suitable occupations according to an individual's assessment and disability. At times, it would provide support to help an individual become independent in many aspects.

I saw him a year later with his mother. He had given up driving and signed up for the local shuttle service, which provided free transportation for special-needs persons. His vision had declined further, and he started learning Braille and received low-vision aids and social services from the Low Vision Center.

What a resilient and remarkable young man.

~ * ~

For individual, family, and caretakers seeking connection and support groups, please check out the References section under Chapter 6, for more information. From my own experience, being part of a support group is essential to help a special-needs person and family sail through the tumultuous time!

Chapter Key Points:

- Retinitis pigmentosa (RP) is a group of genetic disorders.
- The common symptoms of RP are night blindness (difficulty seeing in dim light) and tunnel vision, as if looking through a narrow tube (loss of the peripheral vision).
- The rate of progressive vision loss in RP is unpredictable and varies by individual.
- The primary symptoms of Usher syndrome are deafness or hearing loss and an eye disease called retinitis pigmentosa (RP), which usually results in the patient becoming legally blind by the age of forty.
- Many low-vision devices are available to help patients with RP.
- The advance of cochlear implants may benefit the patient with Usher syndrome to gain sound awareness or hearing.

Chapter 7

"Do I really need more than one pair of glasses?"

The Stories of Computer Glasses, Sports and Work Safety, and Sun Protection

*"**Computer Vision Syndrome**, also referred to as **Digital Eye Strain**, describes a group of eye and vision-related problems that result from prolonged computer, tablet, e-reader and cell phone use. Many individuals experience eye discomfort and vision problems when viewing digital screens for extended periods. The level of discomfort appears to increase with the amount of digital screen use."*

~AOA

"**MY EYES FEEL** like popping out of my eye

sockets at the end of the day."

"My neck and head hurt so much. My chiropractor recommended that I have an eye exam."

"My eyes are so dry. I can't keep my contact lenses on."

"The words on my computer screen come in and out of focus and dance around after a while."

"After work, my distant vision becomes so blurred that I don't see well while driving."

I had heard these kinds of complaints almost daily in recent years. Nowadays, these complaints have even come from elementary-school children. It's alarming and heart-wrenching to hear school kids cry about the intensity of their headaches. At times, I worried that I might miss brain tumors. I've even referred a couple of patients to the neurologist in the past.

Clinically, Computer Vision Syndrome is also called Digital Eye Strain. Because its effect is not only restrained to computer work, it also encompasses all the eye stresses related to smartphones or near-work gadgets, like iPads and other tablets.

YOUR PRECIOUS SIGHT

During the case history, I routinely asked my patients whether they did any computer work. If yes, to save time, I handed the patient a list of ergonomic workspaces recommended by the Occupational Safety and Health Administration (OSHA), and reinforced the pertinence of the 20-20-20 rule: every 20 minutes, look at something 20 feet away for 20 seconds.

At the end of the exam, to explain the function of a pair of computer glasses, my crafted script would be something like this: "When you're working on the computer, the lens in your eyes needs to zoom in, just like when you're taking photos of a close-up object and you need to dial-in the camera lens. When the focusing/accommodative system of your eyes locks in at a near distance for a while, your eyes get fatigued and your body tenses up. Then you have eyestrain and physical pains. The computer glasses are designed to do this work for you, to relieve your focus stress so your eyes don't need to work so hard."

I know it sounds like a long script, but it only took a minute or so to explain. However, I have said it countless times; I was sick of listening to myself. To overcome the broken record, lifeless tone, I had to conjure up some gesticulation and poses, adding a bit of the theatrical element to make my speech intriguing.

This script made a reasonable impact on a person who understood the mechanism of a real camera. However, for some of the new smartphone generation, the concept of "zoom in at the close-up object" was a bit abstract unless they already took physics classes in school. I said it anyway and enforced that "the computer glasses will do the work for you, relieve your eye strain."

I believe it's a disservice to my patients who work on a computer eight hours a day if I don't provide computer glasses and communicate the benefits of them. It's also pertinent to educate them about the function of the antireflective coating and blue light filter add-on for computer glasses. The antireflective coating will reduce glare. The blue light filter will block out most of the harmful rays that can damage the macular cells and potentially increase the risk of macular degeneration. I want my patients to acquire all these facts from me in order to lessen confusion when they face the optician or dispensing staff.

A good friend of mine who lives in Arizona

YOUR PRECIOUS SIGHT

called me from the parking lot outside of an optical store the other day. She said, "I felt like they were like a bunch of car salesmen, pushing me with all the add-ons. They were trying to drain my wallet and suck my blood."

Before ending this section, I dare not forget my dear contact lens patients who spend long hours on the computer.

"Remember to blink. Install non-preservative artificial tears if needed. A pair of computer glasses over contact lenses would help." That's all I say.

~ * ~

"Wearing the right protective eyewear during sports and recreation is a must. Not wearing proper eyewear is like playing basketball barefoot or snow skiing without ski poles. You're just asking for injuries. The right eyewear helps you see clearly, protects your eyes from injury, and helps you play your best."

~ Vision Service Plan (VSP)

"HIS COACH WANTED him to get a pair of

sports glasses," Brian's mother said.

"What happened here?" I pointed to the Band-Aid on the corner of his right eye.

"We signed him up for the soccer league this school year. The ball hit him and broke his glasses. The side-piece scratched the skin. It wasn't too deep," Brian's mother said on his behalf. The small boy was seated on the examination chair with his legs crossed, gazed down.

"Wow! Good thing it didn't scratch his eye." I meant it. The gruesome image of a side-piece (the temple of a frame) stuck into his eyeball, teetering, like a scene in a horror movie, invaded my head and gave me goosebumps. I quickly dismissed it.

"That's why he needs sports glasses. A few kids on his team have them. He's due for an eye exam anyway. We'll just get them with the new prescription."

Brian was in the second grade and had been wearing glasses fulltime for astigmatism since kindergarten.

"You're a caring mother," I said sincerely, glad that I had not shared my disturbing worst-case-scenario thoughts with her.

YOUR PRECIOUS SIGHT

In retrospect, there had been those sports-related eye injuries that had caused a big stir during my years in practice. One of them was a patient hit by a racquetball. The blunt trauma caused a 35-year-old executive an angle closure. The draining system of the eye was shut down due to the injury, which shot his intraocular pressure (IOP) to 60 mmHg (normal IOP ranges from 12-22 mmHg). It was an emergency because an increase of IOP can rapidly damage the optic nerve, the nerve bundle in the eye that transmits information to the brain, and cause vision loss! I worked frantically to control his IOP with assistance from a nearby ophthalmologist, preventing his optic nerve head from experiencing permanent damage due to traumatic glaucoma. It was chaos beyond words. Later on, a small retinal tear affected by the impact of the flying ball was found in that assaulted eye. Fortunately, it did not turn into a full-blown retinal detachment and was repaired with laser surgery.

Note: The angle is referred to the angle between the iris (the colored part of the eye) and the cornea (the clear front window of the eye). This angle is also called the drainage angle; it allows the outflow of fluid in the eye to prevent pressure from building up and leading to glaucoma.

*"**Traumatic glaucoma** is any glaucoma caused by an injury to the eye. This type of glaucoma can occur both immediately after an injury to the eye or years later."*

~Glaucoma Research Foundation

For all sports aficionados, please listen carefully: wear your sports-safety eyewear!

Note: For a glasses frame or goggle to be claimed as official sports eyewear, it must meet the specifications of the American Society for Testing and Materials (ASTM) F803 requirements. Not only do the lenses have to be a durable and high-impact-resistant material, but the frame must be as well, with rubber padding at every point that makes contact with the wearer's face.

For more information, please check out the References section at the back, under Chapter 7.

~ * ~

YOUR PRECIOUS SIGHT

"All too often, when we're working around the house and doing chores that we've done a thousand times before without incident, we forget about the risks we take by not protecting our eyes," said Hugh R. Parry, president and CEO of Prevent Blindness America. "But all it takes is one split-second accident that could damage your vision for a lifetime."

~*Occupational Health & Safety*

A FEW MINUTES before 4 p.m., the entire staff gathered in the front office, chitchatting about turkeys, pumpkin pies, and Black Friday shopping, ready to call it a day. It was Thanksgiving Eve, and our office closed early.

The phone rang.

"Hurry! Go turn on the answering machine," one of our assistants urged.

Too late. Another assistant picked up the receiver instinctively.

"Please hold for a second. Let me ask the doctors," she said to the caller after thirty seconds. She punched the Mute button.

"He said it's an emergency. He thinks

something got into his eye." Her eyes darted between my practice partner-husband, and me. My husband took the receiver.

I tapped on my wristwatch and mouthed at him while he was talking on the phone, reminding him that the kids were flying in in a couple of hours at John Wayne Airport.

He nodded.

"The front door will be locked. The answering machine will be on. Just call me on my cell phone when you get here." Before hanging up, my partner gave the caller his cell phone number.

Somehow, I *knew* he would do so.

About fifteen minutes later, his iPhone rang.

He opened the door and greeted the guy, who had one red eye.

Since all assistants had gone for the day, I sat in my partner's exam room while he took care of Mr. Gonzales, just in case he needed a hand.

Mr. Gonzales was a retired firefighter in his early sixties, at least six feet tall and fit, and had been one of our long-term patients. He enjoyed welding as a hobby and pastime.

YOUR PRECIOUS SIGHT

"We haven't used our fireplace since we bought the house. You know, in Southern California . . . But my wife thought it would be nice to use it for this holiday since the grandkids are coming. I was welding, making a firewood rack and fireguard. I think something flew into my right eye."

"When did it happen?" my husband asked him.

"Last weekend. I washed my eyes right away, it was better, but the irritation didn't go away and seemed to get worse. I thought I'd better get it checked."

My partner whizzed through the case history, visual acuity, and a slit-lamp exam.

"Yeah, a piece of metal is lodged on the cornea, 2mm off the center toward the temple side. When it heals, the scar should not affect your central vision, except at night," he said to the big guy, who kept his eyes as wide as saucers, not daring to blink.

With an eye spud, my partner removed the tiny piece of metal. He also had to use the Alger brush to clean the rust ring in order to avoid further corneal damage and to facilitate fast healing. Afterward, he instilled a couple of antibiotic drops for prophylaxis.

"Wow! That feels so much better. I should have come in sooner. I'm glad I caught you, Doc. I'd hate to sit in the emergency room or have to deal with the pain through our turkey dinner." The patient smiled.

He received a prescription for antibiotic ophthalmic solution to prevent an eye infection from the trauma, and he also got an earful from my partner about using safety eyewear with side shields.

"I always do. It's just one time I forgot to put it on," he said.

Famous last words. We've all heard that before.

Eye safety had always been a real concern, not only at work but at home, for adults and children alike. We had seen kids injured from toys.

According to the American Academy of Ophthalmology's recent eye health statistics, an estimated 2.4 million eye injuries occur in the United States each year. Notably, forty percent of eye injuries happen at home, and ten to twenty percent of injuries will cause temporary

YOUR PRECIOUS SIGHT

or permanent vision loss. Using protective eyewear can prevent ninety percent of all eye injuries.

There is an urgency to promote the awareness of eye safety. Please allow me to quote the following message:

"Prevent Blindness America strongly supports the AAO and the American Society of Ocular Trauma (ASOT) in their recommendation that every household should have at least one pair of American National Standards Institute (ANSI)-approved eyewear. The eyewear should have the Z-87 logo stamped on the frames and can be purchased inexpensively at hardware stores and home building centers."

It's recommended that a set of side shields attached to the safety glasses to prevent the flying objects or small particles from landing and lodging obliquely on the eyeball.

~ * ~

"Most people are aware of how harmful UV radiation is to the skin. However, many may not realize that UV radiation can harm the eyes, and other components

of solar radiation can also affect vision. The longer the eyes are exposed to solar radiation, the greater the risk of developing cataracts or macular degeneration later in life. It is not clear how much exposure to solar radiation will cause damage. Therefore, whenever you spend time outdoors, wear quality sunglasses that offer UV protection and a hat or cap with a wide brim."

~AOA

"**THE PIECES OF** meat in my eyes are growing. They make my eyes look red, like I had too many drinks. They feel sore lately," Jorge complained. He was an ocean lifeguard at Huntington Beach.

"You meant your pterygia?" I knew exactly what he meant.

I reviewed his previous file. Indeed, his pterygia on both nasal sides of his conjunctiva were growing. They were spreading into his corneas. Because of that, his prescription had shown a significant increase in astigmatism.

"I am referring you to a surgeon for an evaluation to see whether it's time to have them surgically removed." I also mentioned that they might regrow after surgery, so it was important to wear UV-protective sunglasses.

Pterygium is also called "surfer's eye." It is a raised, wedged-shaped lump that starts on the sclera (the white part of the eyeball) and can encroach the cornea. Ultraviolet (UV) radiation from the sun and the sandy wind have been believed to be the prime causes for its growth and development.

I am always an enthusiast for advocating wearing sunglasses to protect the eyes from sun damage. Sunglasses are like sunscreen for the eyes. Sun protection is not only for adults but also for children.

At a health fair many years ago, a reporter asked me whether a pair of sunglasses with the darker tint was better for protection of the eyes.

"The color and the density of the tint are not my primary concern," I told him. "The importance is the lenses possessing the ability to block UV lights. As a matter of fact, it's hazardous to wear a pair of sunglasses having no UV blocking function because our pupils enlarge behind the dark-tinted lenses, which would permit a greater amount of harmful radiation to reach the retina."

I want to reiterate (bear with me) that you should not go for inferior-quality sunglasses with poor optics and inadequate UV protection. I don't mean that you should get a pair of designer sunglasses or sacrifice your entire month of grocery money for super-expensive sunglasses. I do suggest a pair of good-quality sunglasses having a sticker or tag indicating that they block 100 percent of UV light with no distortion on the lenses.

Extended exposure to the sun's UV rays has been linked to eye damage, including cataracts, macular degeneration, dry eyes, pingueculae, pterygia, and photokeratitis.

For detailed information about UV radiation and your eyes, please the References section at the back.

So, back to the question:

"Do I really need more than one pair of glasses?" This is a legitimate question, and it comes up often.

With advances in technology, you can find

YOUR PRECIOUS SIGHT

glasses to meet a wide range of eyewear needs. Choices include glasses with photochromatic transition lenses that function as both sunglasses and regular glasses, like the popular SunSensors. Progressive or multifocal lenses are becoming easier to adapt. Polycarbonate lenses are available in a wide variety of designs. You can even find side shields to attach to the temples of your glasses. There's something for everyone! And, in reality, it is not impossible to include all of these features in one pair of glasses.

Notwithstanding, let's imagine having only one pair of shoes to wear all day long and for all activities—working, walking your dog, playing golf or other sports, attending your good friend's wedding, showing up at your mother-in-law's or your boss's birthday party, and so on. That just wouldn't work, would it?

Don't you think your eyes warrant at least as much variety and attention as your feet?

Chapter Key Points:

- Computer Vision Syndrome, also referred to as Digital Eye Strain, is the eye discomfort and vision problems caused by viewing digital screens for extended periods. The level of discomfort appears to increase with the amount of digital screen use.
- The 20-20-20 rule is to lessen digital eyestrain: every 20 minutes, look at something 20 feet away for 20 seconds.
- A pair of computer glasses with antireflective coating can reduce eyestrain. The blue light filter is reported to lessen the incidents of macular degeneration or other eye diseases.
- Wearing the right kind of protective eyewear at home or play can protect your or your child's eyes from injuries.
- For a glasses frame or goggle to be claimed as a "Sports Eyewear," it has to meet the specifications of the American Society for Testing and Materials (ASTM) F803 requirements. Not only do the lenses have to be a durable and high-impact-resistant material, but the frame must be as well, with rubber padding at every point that makes contact

YOUR PRECIOUS SIGHT

with the wearer's face.

- Every household should have at least one pair of American National Standards Institute (ANSI)-approved eyewear. The eyewear should have the Z-87 logo stamped on the frames with side shields.
- The longer the eyes are exposed to UV radiation, the greater the risk of developing cataracts or macular degeneration later in life.
- Sunglasses are like sunscreen for the eyes. Sun protection is not only for adults but also for children.
- A pair of good-quality sunglasses should have a sticker or tag indicating that they block 100 percent of UV light with no distortion on the lenses.

Chapter 8

"I want to get rid of glasses and contact lenses!"

The Stories of Refractive Surgeries

"Most patients are very pleased with the results of their refractive surgery. However, like any other medical procedure, there are risks involved. That's why it is important for you to understand the limitations and possible complications of refractive surgery.... Be cautious about slick advertising and/or deals that sound too good to be true. Remember, they usually are. There is a lot of competition resulting in a great deal of advertising and bidding for your business. Do your homework."

~FDA

"ANOTHER EYE INFECTION!" Trish sighed.

YOUR PRECIOUS SIGHT

Besides her red eye, she looked absolutely fabulous. Dressed in Victoria's Secret *PINK* leggings and a white spaghetti-strap top, the petite woman was tan, slim, and fit.

Three years prior, she had been thirty-five pounds overweight after giving birth to two children, one right after the other. One day she decided to be a triathlete.

When she first told me, I admit I was skeptical. She had never seemed like an athlete to me. Now, she had completed more than a dozen competitions. I saw the posts of her races on Instagram once in a while. I especially liked the ones where her family embraced her when she triumphantly completed the race.

The triathlon she participated in included running, swimming, and cycling. She used to wear monthly planned replacement contact lenses for her moderate myopia (nearsightedness). I switched her to one-day disposables once she was in sports. She told me that the swimming part of the competition was in open water most of the time. I instructed her to discard the contact lenses as soon as she could after swimming, training, or racing, and then rinse her eyes with non-preservative artificial tears afterward.

Races were challenging because swimming was not the last event most of the time. Even though she wore swimming goggles, she still got punctate keratitis and conjunctivitis from time to time.

"I've been thinking about laser surgery to get rid of the contact lenses. I'm ready for it," Trish said.

There were a few refractive surgery options for her prescription.

Refractive surgery is a procedure to correct refractive errors, which can be myopia (nearsightedness), hyperopia (farsightedness), astigmatism (mostly referring to the American-football-shaped eyeball), and presbyopia (usually occurs after forty years old).

With advances in technology, the diligence of clinical researchers, and constant fine-tuning of surgical procedures, there are many options for refractive surgeries nowadays, and they are continuously evolving. To name a few, there are LASIK, PRK, RLE and PRELEX, Intacs, Phakic Intraocular Lens Implants, and LRI.

"You may not participate in the race during

the healing period after the surgery. To avoid adverse effects, it can be months—and that's a conservative estimate," I told Trish while treating her red eye during that visit.

We referred her to a surgeon we trusted, and she went in for a thorough evaluation. She had the laser-assisted in-situ keratomileusis (LASIK) procedure done a month later.

At her one-day post-op follow-up, she saw 20/20 in each eye. She was elated!

In our office, after determining whether a patient was the proper candidate, with rational motivation and expectations, we provided handouts and discussed the options and the surgeons' profiles in order for patients to make an informed decision.

We only referred patients to surgeons who had proven skills and experience, updated instrumentations, and ethics, with unbeatable success rates. They might not have been the cheapest; however, they were the ones we trusted with our hearts.

For more information, please check out the References section at the back, under Chapter 8.

DR. EICHIN CHANG-LIM

~ * ~

MY BEST FRIEND, Jennifer, laced her fingers and bowed her head. I sat next to her, silently praying. We were in the waiting room of an outpatient surgical center. Her daughter, Jannet, had undergone a refractive surgery called phakic intraocular lens implants (ICL). The surgeon was very experienced and reputable in this field; we had done co-management with him for over a decade. We had all the confidence in him. Nevertheless, it was a surgery.

I had known Jannet since she was a baby; it almost seemed as if I grew old with her. She started wearing glasses at six years old for her nearsightedness. During her teenage years, the prescription accelerated rapidly. When she entered UC Berkeley, she had -10 diopters of myopia.

In the summer after her first year of medical school, I referred her to the above-mentioned trusted surgeon to have a refractive surgery evaluation. Her myopic measurement was -13.50 diopters, and her prescription was unstable. The goal was to obtain the surgeon's opinion regarding her options. We learned that her prescription was too high and that her cornea was too thin for the conventional LASIK procedure. Another concern was that her corneal topography, a computerized image with a three-dimensional map of the surface curvature of the cornea, revealed some warpage. Her cornea distortion could be due to her long hours of wearing contact lenses.

During her last two years of medical school, we monitored her prescription and were convinced that it had stabilized. She matched to a prestigious hospital for her residency program and was one month away from receiving her medical degree. Considering the demanding hours and vigorous training she would face in the upcoming years, Jannet decided to undergo refractive surgery so that she would not have to fuss with contact lenses.

A phakic intraocular lens implant, also called implantable Collamer lens (ICL), is a biocompatible plastic lens inserted behind the patient's pupil or attached to the iris (the colored part of the eye) without provoking any insult to a patient's natural lens. This procedure incurs minimal corneal insults, and the implanted lens is removable. However, the surgeon needs to perform the laser iridotomy, a procedure to open a hole at the peripheral iris with a laser to ensure no blockage of the fluid drainage, one week before the actual surgery to prevent the potential occurrence of glaucoma. (More information regarding glaucoma is included in a later chapter.)

The door at the far corner of the room opened, and the surgeon and Jannet emerged sooner than we'd expected. Both were smiling. My friend and I exhaled sighs of relief.

Not long after leaving the surgical center, though, Jannet complained about a headache. I was the volunteer driver; Jennifer held Jannet's hand and comforted her. However, Jannet soon started to cry.

"My head is going to split open," Jannet said between sobs, squeezing her temples with her palms. She began to wail. I knew this girl. She was always levelheaded and well composed.

Something is not right!

Sensing the emergency, I drove mother and daughter to the surgeon's office at once. One of the surgeon's associates attended to Jannet in haste. We were all aware of what was happening. Indeed, the Goldmann tonometry—an instrument to measure intraocular pressure (IOP)—read her right eye's IOP as 55 mmHg. Normal IOP is 12-22 mmHg. Prolonged elevated IOP can damage the optic nerve head and lead to permanent visual impairment. Time was of the essence!

All the treatments to lower the IOP were initiated in no time, including instilling glaucoma drops and digitally massaging the eye to promote the drainage of the extra fluid induced during the surgery. Since she'd had laser iridotomy one week before the ICL surgery, the fluid drained out from the anterior chamber of her eye swiftly, and her IOP was soon under control.

Jannet's headache subsided once the IOP dropped to the normal range. We were in the clinic for several hours to ensure her IOPs were normal and stable. We monitored her recovery closely for one week.

Jannet's best correctable vision was 20/20 in each eye one month later.

"I have never seen so well in my life. Everything looks so much sharper. I feel much safer driving," she remarked.

Before refractive surgery, her best correctable

vision had fluctuated between 20/25 and 20/30 in each eye, either with contact lenses or spectacles. Despite the nerve-racking episode right after the surgery, she was delighted with the results.

~ * ~

Before leaving this chapter, let me share the quote with a profound message with you:

"The bottom line is that you only have one pair of eyes, and your vision is your most precious sense. It is important to carefully consider your options when it comes to refractive surgery: your surgeon; the philosophy of the practice; the quality of the support staff. All of these are very important decisions for what is truly 'the visual event of a lifetime.'"

> ~ *Flaum Eye Institute at the University of Rochester*

Please note that refractive surgery can be an adverse procedure for some people. Please find out who should not have it done. Check out the References sections at the back under Chapter 8.

YOUR PRECIOUS SIGHT

Chapter Key Points:

- Like any other medical procedure, there are risks involved with refractive surgeries. There are many options for refractive surgeries nowadays, and they are continuously evolving. The procedure should be customized individually. Keep in mind that each technique has advantages and disadvantages. Do your homework!
- In general, the majority of people who have refractive eye surgery achieve the desired vision, which works well for most activities. However, most people still eventually need glasses for driving at night or for near-vision.
- Your vision must be stable before considering refractive surgery.
- Having healthy corneas is imperative for refractive surgeries. You have to completely stop wearing your contact lenses and switch to glasses for at least a few weeks before your refractive surgery, because contact lenses compromise the integrity of the cornea.
- If considering refractive surgery, a good starting point when choosing an eye surgeon

is to talk with the eyecare professional you know and trust.

- People who **should not** have refractive surgery are those with the following: conditions that impair wound healing, like autoimmune or connective tissue diseases; active eye diseases, like severe dry-eye, chronic eyelid infection, or distorted cornea; Keratoconus (cone-shaped corneas); a previous herpes simplex eye infection; or those taking certain drugs. Be sure to communicate with your doctor about your medical, ocular, and drug-intake history.

Chapter 9

"When I move my eyes, they hurt!"

The Stories of Multiple Sclerosis

*"**Multiple sclerosis** (MS) involves an immune-mediated process in which an abnormal response of the body's immune system is directed against the central nervous system (CNS). The CNS is made up of the brain, spinal cord and optic nerves. A vision problem is the first symptom of MS for many people. Fortunately, the prognosis is good for recovery from many vision problems associated with MS."*

~National Multiple Sclerosis Society

WHEN I WALKED into the exam room, Amanda barely looked up. That was so uncharacteristic of her. She was thirty-three years old and owned a successful floral shop a few blocks from the office. I'd just seen her and her husband not long ago for their annual exams. Her husband worked in an aerospace company with good vision benefits. She had low myopia (nearsightedness) and only wore glasses for night driving.

Normally, her vivacious personality could light up a room, but not on that particular day. She was sluggish, like a saggy balloon. I was concerned.

"Is everything all right?" I asked her.

"Not really," she mumbled, her droopy body shifting tentatively in the chair. She looked defeated.

"For last two days, I could not see well with my right eye. When I move my eyes sideways, they hurt. Like this way." She demonstrated it by moving her eyes and then let out a quiet, "Ouch." I observed her carefully as she continued.

"And when I arranged the flowers today, I noticed that the color seemed dimmer through my right eye. I also seemed to lose strength in my fingers. They feel numb, and I keep dropping things. I guess I'm just exhausted."

YOUR PRECIOUS SIGHT

While listening to her, I sensed a slur in her speech and took note of it. I recalled reading an article from an optometric journal several nights before about the signs and symptoms of multiple sclerosis (MS). Amanda's symptoms sounded awfully familiar.

Do not jump to conclusions too soon, I reminded myself. I needed to gather information first. In the article, optic neuritis was the cause of all these ocular symptoms, so I focused on the relevant tests.

When I did the red cap test, Amanda reported that the redness when looking through her right eye was less saturated. She expressed it as 60 cents versus one dollar, which meant the redness perceived through her right eye was 60% of the saturation as when looking through her left eye. The red cap test is one of the tests to assess the integrity and symmetry of optic nerve function between two eyes. Most of the time, the red caps on the dilating drops were used for this test. A neuro-ophthalmological defect will desaturate the color perception.

Her eye muscle movements were jerky when she looked sideways. The best correctable vision was 20/60 on the right eye, which had been 20/20 one month ago. The digital retinal photography showed a swollen, pale optic nerve head on the right eye.

I debated whether I should convey the findings and announce the diagnosis of MS to her. However, I refrained from doing so.

"Amanda, I'd like to refer you to a neurologist for a multiple sclerosis evaluation. Do not lose sleep over this. Avoid taking hot showers or hot baths until you see him. Try to stay as cool as you can."

Heat is reported to exacerbate the MS symptoms.

A couple of weeks later, I received a letter from the neurologist. Indeed, after a battery of tests, including an MRI, Amanda was diagnosed with MS.

According to research and reports, the early diagnosis and treatment of MS have a positive impact on a patient's quality of life, slowing the progression of the disease and extending the patient's life span.

Please check out the References section at the back under Chapter 9, to learn about how early diagnosis of MS benefits the quality of life.

YOUR PRECIOUS SIGHT

~ * ~

MY ASSISTANT INFORMED me that Amanda called earlier to let us know that her husband would be home late to give her a ride. It had been five years since Amanda's MS diagnosis.

I was in my office going through some paperwork and heard the conversations.

"I like this long walk. It helps me add steps to my daily goal."

"What's your daily goal?" my assistant asked Amanda while walking with her down the hallway.

"3,000 steps. My Fitbit doesn't let me get away." Amanda laughed. Wobbly, she held onto her walker and went one step at a time. Her husband trailed behind.

I stood by the exam room door, watching them slowly approach. She was my last patient; there was no hurry.

I was filled with admiration. My eyes burned, but I held back my tears. The disease had taken a toll on her; now, she relied on a walker. There were several types of MS. She had the aggressive or progressive kind, she told me.

"I have trouble seeing these days. Not the kind of blurry like when MS attacks. It's like looking out a window through a lace curtain." Amanda explained her trouble once she was situated in the exam chair. "I need to see good so that I can chat online with my friends," she added.

"Oh, what sites are you usually on?" I was intrigued.

"I chat on Facebook and Twitter, mainly. I take flower pictures with my iPhone whenever I can and post them on Instagram. I like to talk to my MS friends. We talk a lot. We joke about how to get to the toilet fast to avoid an incident. Stuff like that," Amanda said with a smile.

"She's more social media savvy than I am," her husband chipped in.

I checked her eyes. The slit lamp exam revealed posterior subcapsular cataracts in both eyes. Posterior subcapsular cataracts are opaque areas beneath the back membrane of the natural lens, one of the possible side effects in patients who take a systemic steroid.

I communicated the findings to Amanda,

and she admitted that she had undergone heavy doses of steroid treatment in the midst of her last two MS attacks.

"My MS specialist warned me about the side effects of the steroid, including cataracts," she said, her voice calm.

"Let me refer you to a cataract surgeon," I said to her. "He can restore your vision so you can chat online in no time." I briefly went through the process of cataract surgery with her.

I followed up with her after the surgery. Her vision was 20/25 in her right eye and 20/20 in her left eye.

We were both pleased with the outcome. Her fighting spirit continued. It's wonderful that she found support groups online and could enjoy her life, despite the affliction.

I cheered for her!

Furthermore, Amanda taught me that being part of a supportive group is vital when coping with chronic conditions like MS.

I have found a few support groups for MS patients to get connected. Please check out the References section at the back, under Chapter 9.

DR. EICHIN CHANG-LIM

~ * ~

MS is not the only autoimmune disorder to exhibit ocular manifestations. Other autoimmune diseases can also cause ocular symptoms like dry eyes, red eyes, light sensitivity, pain, and vision change, or even vision loss. It is not uncommon that an eye doctor is the first person who suspects the disease and initiates prompt testing that leads to the diagnose of the disease.

The list of autoimmune diseases that affect the ocular system includes, but is not limit to, rheumatoid arthritis (RA), juvenile rheumatoid arthritis, Sjögren's syndrome, the seronegative spondyloarthropathies, systemic lupus erythematosus, multiple sclerosis, giant cell arteritis, Graves' disease, Behcet's disease, psoriasis, Reiter's syndrome, type 1 diabetes, ulcerative colitis , Crohn's disease, and uveitis.

Ultimately, the control and treatment of the diseases require multiple professionals' ongoing open communication and collaborative efforts.

YOUR PRECIOUS SIGHT

Chapter Key Points:

- For many people, a vision problem is the first symptom of MS. The vision problems can be blurry or double vision, loss of vision or color contrast, or pain while moving the eye.
- Fortunately, the prognosis for recovery from many vision problems associated with MS is good.
- MS symptoms vary individually. The most common early signs of MS include vision problems, tingling and numbness, pains and spasms, weakness or fatigue, balance problems or dizziness, bladder and bowel issues, sexual dysfunction, cognitive problems, and depression.
- According to research and reports, early diagnosis and treatment of MS have a positive impact on a patient's quality of life, slowing the progression of the disease and extending the patient's life span.
- A posterior subcapsular cataract is one of the possible side effects in patients who take systemic steroids.
- Besides MS, other autoimmune disorders impacting the health of the eyes and vision

are Behcet's disease, lupus, psoriasis, Reiter's syndrome, rheumatoid arthritis (RA), Sjogren's syndrome, thyroid diseases, type 1 diabetes, ulcerative colitis, Crohn's disease, uveitis, and others.

Chapter 10

"I am under so much stress."

The Stories of Eye Twitching, Central Serous Retinopathy, and Hysterical Blindness

---

"An eyelid twitch is a general term for spasms of the eyelid muscles. These spasms happen without your control. The eyelid may repeatedly close (or nearly close) and reopen…The most common things that make the muscle in your eyelid twitch are fatigue, stress, and caffeine."

~U.S. National Library of Medicine

JOHN'S EYES WERE glued to his iPad as I entered the room. From my angle of view, it looked like he was on iBook.

"A fun read?" I asked him. "Some kind of thriller or suspense?"

He lifted his head and leaned back. "Fun read? NO! Much more frightening than a thriller, though. I'm afraid my professor is going to kill me in this class." His eyes were bloodshot.

John had been our patient since high school and had worn contact lenses for several years. A few months ago, he was enthusiastic about his acceptance into law school. Based on the front office schedule, he was here for a six-month contact lens follow-up.

Instead of jumping right into the exam, I struck up a conversation with him. "So, what classes are you taking?"

"All the fundamental classes . . . Criminal Law, Civil Procedure, Contracts, Torts. They're sort of interesting. It's just so much reading. Too much! The legal research writing assignments have been challenging too. I'm not the best writer." He sighed.

Why are his eyes red? While listening to his rambling, I scrutinized those brown-red eyes. I did not detect any discharge or mucus. John was unshaven and looked exhausted but not in pain.

He continued. "I called this morning for a contact lens follow-up. My real problem is that

YOUR PRECIOUS SIGHT

my eye has been twitching for two days. It's not painful, just twitching. It's annoying and disturbing my concentration."

"Give me a big smile," I said to him. A grin broke out on his fatigue face.

No facial spasms were discerned. No Bell's Palsy (also known as facial palsy).

I went through the contact lens follow-up exam. With contact lenses, his vision was 20/20 minus a few letters for each eye. The over-refraction (the power needed with his contact lenses on) was plano for each eye, which indicated that his contact lens prescription was correct. Furthermore, there was no evidence of any abnormality except for injected conjunctiva (red eye).

"Your eyes are red," I commented as I pushed away the slit lamp.

"I realize that. I've been sleep deprived. Red Bull is my salvation. Getting through this semester is my resolution. Next week's final is my destination." He slumped back in the chair.

"I think that accounts for your eye twitching. Stress can do a lot to your body." I instructed John to wear glasses instead of contact lenses until the final was over.

Moreover, I gave him the following regimen: apply a warm compress on his eyelids to relax the muscles, use non-preservative artificial tears periodically to avoid dry eyes, get adequate sleep, and cut back the caffeine, especially the energy drinks like Red Bull.

"Law school is brutal, especially the first semester. Take a deep breath," I said. "You can do it."

Three years later, John graduated from law school and passed the bar exam.

~ * ~

*"**Central serous chorioretinopathy, commonly referred to as CSC**, is a condition in which fluid accumulates under the retina, causing a serous (fluid-filled) detachment and vision loss. The causes of CSC are not fully understood. It is thought that any systemic exposure to a corticosteroid drug can bring about or worsen CSC. Corticosteroids are found in allergy nose sprays and anti-inflammatory skin creams available over the counter and are often prescribed to treat a variety of medical conditions. An association has also been made between CSC and patients with emotional*

YOUR PRECIOUS SIGHT

distress and/or Type A personalities. It is possible that the body produces natural corticosteroids in times of stress that may trigger CSC in an individual prone to this condition."

~American Society of Retina Specialists

IT IS NOT an overstatement that 2008 was a perturbing year. An undercurrent of fear rattled the rich, the poor, and everyone in between. Almost every day, patients reported that they had lost their jobs, houses, or both. Their insurance had been or was about to be terminated. Even the most protected of citizens—schoolteachers—were receiving pink slips. Government-sponsored vision care benefits were drastically trimmed.

In the midst of that summer, 35-year-old Travis showed up in my exam chair. I barely recognized him. The last time I had seen him was five years prior. At that time, he had been gleeful and confident. He had just quit his retail job to become a day trader; he even proudly proclaimed himself an investor then. Nevertheless, that summer day in 2008, he was bedraggled from head to toe and gazing blankly into space. He resembled someone's grandfather in the early stages of dementia.

"My vision has been blurred and weird in my left eye for three days," Travis murmured.

He denied any medical issues in the case history. Over the course of the comprehensive exam, he mumbled intermittently and shared his devastating conundrum:

He had done remarkably well during his first two years of day trading; he had been able to use the gains from the stock market to purchase a 12-unit apartment complex with a low down payment in the Newport Beach area. As the housing market accelerated, he took out a second mortgage to trade in the stock market. Both markets had betrayed him. His apartment complex was foreclosed upon, and he scrambled to fulfill the margin calls on his brokerage account.

I felt his profound pain; however, I could not find any appropriate words to comfort him. I just let him vent.

On the fundus photography, I found the answer for his vision complaint. He had the condition called central serous retinopathy (CSR), aka Central Serous Chorioretinopathy (CSC).

YOUR PRECIOUS SIGHT

"CSC is a condition in which fluid accumulates under the retina, causing a serous (fluid-filled) detachment and vision loss," according to the American Society of Retina Specialists.

For more information, please check out the References section at the back, under Chapter 10.

In an article in *verywell Health* magazine, Troy Bedinghaus, OD, said, "CSR is sometimes referred to as idiopathic serous chorioretinopathy because the direct cause is not known. There is a lot of controversy in the medical community as to why some people develop the disease; a common recurring theme seems to be stress, and the condition seems to occur when stress levels are high in a person's life. People who take oral steroids are at a slightly higher risk of developing the disease. Lack of sleep also seems to play a role."

To know more about CSR, please check out the References section at the back, under Chapter 10.

Travis clenched his jaw and wrung his hands

as I conveyed these findings to him. When I told him that stress could affect our body and vision, he gave me a wry smile, responded, "Tell me about it. I've had the nagging headaches and stomachaches for some time."

In spite of its nature of being a self-limiting disease with a good prognosis, I always referred a patient with CSR to a trusted retinal specialist for a second opinion. I gave Travis the necessary referral paperwork.

"Also, you should see your primary physician for your headaches and stomachaches," I told him.

"I don't have health care insurance." He emitted a fake laugh. Unsteadily, he stood up and dragged himself out of the exam room.

I haven't seen him since. Nevertheless, he pops into my head occasionally, as both housing and stock markets have rebounded in recent years.

~ * ~

"*Conversion disorder is a mental condition in which a person has blindness, paralysis, or other nervous system (neurologic) symptoms that*

YOUR PRECIOUS SIGHT

cannot be explained by medical evaluation."

~MedlinePlus
(U.S. National Library of Medicine)

"**WELCOME TO THE** office," I said to Savanna, a new patient.

"I have vision insurance under my mom, and I want to use it before my birthday," Savanna explained. Her twenty-sixth birthday was approaching in three weeks. Under the Affordable Care Act, her benefit would be terminated shortly.

On her patient information form, she marked "negative" in all areas. She was unemployed.

She seemed timid. I endeavored to find a subject to break the ice, like the beautiful weather. Then, a lightbulb turned on.

"Happy early birthday," I said, smiling at her.

"I just wanted to make sure my eyes are okay."

I sensed her disquiet, so I probed gently. "Anything about your eyes or your health you want to share with me?"

During our ensuing conversation, she conveyed to me that she'd been diagnosed with hysterical blindness, a form of conversion disorder, two years before, in Chicago. She lost her vision completely for three days when she went through a personal tragedy. She regained her vision after hospitalization and psychiatric treatment. She admitted she was still taking Paxil, an antidepressant, even though she refused to mark it on the patient information form.

I did the comprehensive exam and took digital retinal photos of her eyes. Except for mild myopia (nearsightedness), she had no other signs of ocular concerns. I prescribed her a pair of glasses with transition lenses. She was informed that the antidepressant could cause sunlight sensitivity and dry eyes. I also assured her that her eye health was perfect.

Savanna was happy to be able to use her vision benefits in time.

~ * ~

Personally, I have experienced stomachaches on stressful days. As a health care provider, I fully understand the psychosomatic symptoms, and how emotional distress manifests as physical symptoms. My ways of defusing stress and despondency have been listening to classical music, dance aerobics, and weightlifting. They work magic on me.

There is no shame about having depression. It's essential to deal with the underlying emotional and psychological issues before they take a toll on a person's physical health. Since our eyes are an integral part of our body, our emotions can have a tremendous impact on our vision.

For more information on Conversion Disorder, please check out the References section at the back, under Chapter 10.

YOUR PRECIOUS SIGHT

Chapter Key Points:

- Eyelid twitch is a general term for spasms of the eyelid muscles. The most common things that trigger twitching in the muscle in your eyelid are fatigue, stress, and caffeine.
- A warm compress can ease the eyelid twitching.
- The exact cause of central serous retinopathy (CSR) is still debatable. The condition, in which the fluid accumulates under the retina, causing a serous detachment and vision loss, seems to occur most often in people with high stress levels and a lack of sleep.
- Hysterical blindness is a form of conversion disorder. The exact cause of conversion disorder is uncertain. However, researchers have reported that it is a mental condition in which a person is under great stress or experiencing emotional trauma, which leads to temporary blindness or paralysis that cannot be explained through a medical evaluation.
- Psychosomatic symptoms refer to the way emotional distress manifests as physical symptoms. It is critical to managing the underlying issues.

Chapter 11

"Did my eyes tell you I am on drugs?"

The Stories of How Substance Abuse and Smoking Affect the Eyes

"Drug and alcohol abuse can produce a variety of ocular and neuro-ophthalmic side effects. Drug abuse can lead to unusual ocular disorders. Legal substances, when used in manners for which they have not been prescribed, can also have devastating ophthalmic consequences."

~NIH

YEARS AGO, I did my internship at the VA hospital in downtown Los Angeles. It was a fantastic training ground for students, because we had opportunities to see a variety of cases, especially those so-called "unusual" ones. I encountered many respectful veterans during that rotation. However, there was one in particular who stuck in my head, even after all these years.

He was in his midforties, with unremarkable medical and ocular history. In his bitter voice, he told me he had been in the Vietnam War. I vividly recall his gaunt face, faded jeans, and his Lakers T-shirt and cap. It was basketball season, and we talked about the Lakers game a little. The Lakers had been playing remarkably well for several years in a row. Everyone talked about it! He was pleasant and cooperative as the exam progressed.

After dilating his eyes and performing the binocular indirect ophthalmoscopy (BIO), I was bewildered by the tiny glistening crystalline-like refracting particles surrounding the macular area—the small central portion on the back of the eye responsible for sharp, central vision—in both eyes. They were not brilliant like Christmas lights; they appeared more like minute, radiant stars in a faraway galaxy, the kind you see on a clear night.

They were *fascinating*! They did not look like exudates from the diabetic retinopathy.

YOUR PRECIOUS SIGHT

At the time, the fundus camera was not widely used. Since I did not have a diagnosis for the case, I drew it out, described the findings on the patient's exam form, and presented them to my staff doctor.

"Go back and ask him if he has been on recreational drugs," my staff doctor commented after looking at what I'd written down.

When I did so, the veteran's jaw dropped, and his eyebrows hiked up. "My eyes tell you I was on drugs?"

After I informed the staff doctor about his response, she came to the room to talk to him and obtained his permission to let the other five students take turns viewing the back of his eyes. He sat up straight and gracefully endured all the bright ophthalmoscope lights shining on his wide-open pupils. At the conclusion of his visit, the staff doctor explained to him what those tiny, gleaming refractive particles were and advised him to cease using recreational drugs.

"Make this your weekly case report," the staff doctor said to me later on.

So, the diagnosis, in this case, was Talc Retinopathy. "Talc is an innate mineral used as filler in certain recreational drugs such as methylphenidate hydrochloride, heroin, and cocaine. Talc cannot dissolve in blood, so the mineral becomes embolic."

Emboli is the plural of *embolus*, which means something that travels through the bloodstream, lodges in a blood vessel, and blocks it. Through the years, I had read several case studies in various journals reporting how Talc Retinopathy permanently damaged a person's eyesight and caused blindness. If we see talc particles deposited on the retina, we can confidently assume that they have lodged elsewhere in the person's vascular system, like the lung or brain.

Our eyes are like a mirror that candidly reflects much about a person's hidden history—past or present.

Please check out the References section at the back, under Chapter 11. There's an article I'd like to share with you. In it, the authors "systematically evaluate each part of the visual pathways and discuss how individual drugs may affect them."

~ * ~

YOUR PRECIOUS SIGHT

"Smoking is as bad for your eyes as it is for the rest of your body."

~NEI

"DO YOU SMOKE?"

Even though I could plainly see the pack of cigarettes protruding from the patient's front pocket, I still asked the question.

I had two brothers who were heavy smokers. Even my subtlest objections about their smoking would ruin a good conversation instantly. I knew how hard they had tried to quit. I could almost hear my patient yelling, "Stop bugging me about my smoking!" followed by an exasperated sigh. Smoking is definitely not a habit you can easily shake off.

I recall one day in the human anatomy lab when our instructor directed us to gather around two cadavers, both of which had their lungs exposed. As the formaldehyde thwacked our nostrils and burned our eyes, we could unmistakably identify which one had been a smoker and which one had not. The smoker's lungs were coated black with heavy tar! The striking visual impact motivated a few of my tobacco-devoted classmates to kick the habit.

It is every healthcare provider's obligation to inquire about a patient's smoking habit. Not only do we have to ask, but we also have to document it. Almost everyone is aware of the hazardous effects of smoking on the body, but not everyone has a clear idea of what it does to our eyes.

The fact is, the eyes are an integrated part of the body; everything affecting our body affects our eyes as well. Studies show smoking increases the risk of age-related macular degeneration, cataracts, glaucoma, diabetic retinopathy, uveitis, and dry eye syndrome.

The harmful effects of smoking can damage the visual system of a fetus during a woman's pregnancy. Besides other serious health problems, they cause infant eye disorders such as strabismus and underdevelopment of the optic nerve, which can lead to blindness in affected children.

Take a look at the WHO brochure regarding tobacco packaging. Scroll down to pages four and five to see the images. They are gripping and provocative, in my opinion. Do you think they would make an impact on the public,

YOUR PRECIOUS SIGHT

especially smokers?

Please check out the References section at the back for more information. You'll find them under Chapter 11.

Chapter Key Points:

- Almost all abused substances can have negative effects on the eyes.
- "Talc is an innate mineral used as filler in certain recreational drugs such as methylphenidate hydrochloride, heroin, and cocaine. Talc cannot dissolve in blood, so the mineral becomes embolic." If drug abuse continues, the particles can enlarge, lodge in the blood vessels, and block the blood flow in many parts of the body, like the lungs or brain. In the eye, this can induce ocular complications, such as retinal artery occlusion (a blockage in one of the small arteries that carry blood to the retina) and optic nerve ischemia (blood does not flow properly to the optic nerve), which can lead to severe progressive vision loss and eventually blindness.
- The link between smoking and sight loss is as strong as the link between smoking and lung cancer.
- Addiction and drug abuse harm nearly every part of the body, and the eyes are no exception. Eyes are an integrated part of the body.

YOUR PRECIOUS SIGHT

- Studies show smoking increases the risk of age-related macular degeneration, cataracts, glaucoma, diabetic retinopathy, uveitis, and dry eye syndrome.

Chapter 12

"I'm seeing a curtain coming down in my eyes."

The Stories of Retinal Detachments (RD)

"The retina is the light-sensitive layer of tissue that lines the inside of the eye and sends visual messages through the optic nerve to the brain. When the retina detaches, it is lifted or pulled from its normal position. If not promptly treated, **retinal detachment** *can cause permanent vision loss. In some cases, there may be small areas of the retina that are torn. These areas, called retinal tears or retinal breaks, can lead to retinal detachment."*

~NEI

"**CAN YOU SEE** my brother?" my assistant,

YOUR PRECIOUS SIGHT

Jan, asked me as I prepared to call it a day. It was Friday, nearly 6 p.m. *I want to go home!*

"Why? Is it something urgent?" I asked. I thought about fabricating a believable excuse to defer him till the next morning since I worked through the weekend.

"I think he has retinal detachment." Jan looked concerned.

She had my attention. "What makes you think so?"

"I heard you tell patients about the signs of retinal detachment. He's in the reception area. Can you see him?"

"Of course!" There was no way I could turn him away.

Jan asked me whether she should do pre-testing first.

"Just autorefractor and NCT," I replied. The autorefractor would give a rough estimate of his eyewear prescription, and the Non-Contact Tonometer (NCT) would check his intraocular pressure.

Jan's brother, James, was a 43-year-old self-employed house painter. He'd never had an eye exam before. The autorefractor reading showed he was slightly farsighted with little astigmatism. I glanced at the patient information form; he had marked all negatives on his medical history. My first impression was that he was not in the high-risk category to have retinal detachment.

He was about 5 feet 8 and fit, his pants and tennis shoes stained with splashed paint. Apparently he'd come directly from work.

All pleasantries were omitted. I cut right to the chase once he was seated in my exam room.

"I see a curtain coming down in my right eye. It's driving me crazy," James said, his brows furrowed.

"When did you first experience that?"

"It started last weekend. I also see flashing lights. It's weird."

"Last weekend? And you just came in now?" I almost fell off my chair. I suppressed the surge of anguish bubbling up within me. Instead of reprimanding him for being ignorant, I took a deep breath and proceeded to my next question, my voice calm.

"Anything happened before that?"

"Nothing, really. Well . . . I was organizing

my garage and banged my head on a low shelf. My head hurt, but not my eye. I thought it would go away in a couple of days," he grumbled, a bit defensive.

I checked his eyes with the slit lamp to make sure there were no abnormal findings in the anterior segment and proceeded to dilate his eyes promptly.

It was an excruciating thirty minutes of waiting for his eyes to be fully dilated. Jan was right; her brother had a tear in his right eye's superior retina with a full-blown retinal detachment, and it was encroaching on the central fundus. The macula—the area responsible for central vision—was still on!

It was almost 7 p.m., but my internal voice spoke loudly to me. *We need to save the macula. This is an emergency. Sending him to a hospital ER is not an option.*

I called Dr. Jarus, the retinal specialist. The telephone exchange service answered. The lady told me she'd page Dr. Jarus. A few minutes later, he called back. As luck would have it, he was on call that weekend.

Dr. Jarus made arrangements to have James checked in at his affiliated hospital immediately.

He ordered the patient to lie flat until he saw him the next day, in the hope that gravity would pull the retina down to prevent further detachment.

The retinal specialist did the scleral buckling procedure on James the next morning. He called me later that day about the surgery.

"The patient is lucky that his macula was spared. His best corrected vision on that eye should be affected only minimally. The outcome would be different if he'd waited any longer."

James was under the retinal specialist's care for one year to ensure that no traction occurred to induce further retinal tears or holes during the healing process. He returned to our office for routine eye exams after that. I told him he needed to be seen in haste if anything appeared unusual.

"Do not tough it out with a six-pack of beer." He laughed as I said it.

~ * ~

"A sudden increase in floaters, possibly accompanied by light flashes or peripheral (side) vision loss,

YOUR PRECIOUS SIGHT

could indicate a retinal detachment. A retinal detachment occurs when any part of the retina, the eye's light-sensitive tissue, is lifted or pulled from its normal position at the back wall of the eye. Those who experience a sudden increase in floaters, flashes of light in peripheral vision, or a loss of peripheral vision should have an eye care professional examine their eyes as soon as possible."

~NEI

"**YOUR NEXT PATIENT** is a walk-in. She is on her lunch hour and in a rush." I was about to leave for my lunch, but my assistant handed me Blair's chart. Blair, a 24-year-old, worked as a teller in a nearby bank. She had been one of my contact lenses patients since junior high.

I entered the exam room, and Blair quickly dropped her smartphone into her oversized purse. At once, I noticed she was wearing her glasses. I knew she hated wearing them. She called them "Coke-bottle glasses" because the lenses were thick, like the bottom of a Coke bottle. She had 7 diopters of nearsightedness (myopia).

"How is life treating you?" I asked.

DR. EICHIN CHANG-LIM

"Busy, but okay."

"Running out of contact lenses?" I said as I looked into her eyes.

"I don't know if I'm having a migraine attack like last time or something else. I'm seeing flashing lights. I remember you told me that if I saw flashing lights or unusual floaters, I needed to come in right away." She spelled out her concerns without answering my question directly.

"In that case, I need to dilate your eyes. You will have difficulty seeing well at work, and I don't want you to drive right afterward."

"It's all right. I'll call my supervisor. You just need to write me a note. I can call my mom or sister to pick me up."

While we were waiting for her eyes to dilate, I grabbed a quick bite, and she made phone calls.

Since she had light-colored eyes that responded to the dilating agents relatively fast, her pupils were wide open when I checked on her twenty minutes later.

The binocular indirect ophthalmoscopy (BIO) reveal a small fresh tear at the superior temple at around eleven o'clock in her left eye.

YOUR PRECIOUS SIGHT

The location of the tear was a threat, so I referred Blair to the retinal specialist right away. He was able to use a laser to seal the hole on the same day.

She had no problem resuming the use of her contact lenses shortly afterward. However, she understood that the degree of her nearsightedness positioned her in a higher risk group for retinal detachment.

~ * ~

The following analogy is a routine part of patient education. I communicate with my patients at the end of the exam, especially for those who are at higher risk of retinal detachment, such as those with nearsightedness (myopia), astigmatism greater than -4.00 diopters, diabetes, and people with prior cataract surgery or injury. The analogy is not perfect but helps patients grasp the idea easier.

Our eyes are like a sealed chamber filled with fluid. Wallpaper, which is embedded with electrical wires, is attached to the walls. Nearsighted (myopic) eyeballs tend to be elongated. It's as if the wallpaper is stretched and thinned and, therefore, more prone to tearing or breaking. Incidents like a sudden external impact or the effects of diabetes can weaken the bond between wall and wallpaper. When a tear occurs, the wallpaper pulls away from the wall, triggering the electrical system embedded in the wall. That's why patients see a flashing light.

If the hole or tear in the wallpaper is detected early, it's much easier to seal it with a glue gun (laser or freezing). Otherwise, the fluid seeps into the hole, the wallpaper drags away from the wall, and the collapse will lead to a full-blown detachment. In that case, the patient's eyesight is in jeopardy, and the repairing/treatment procedure is complicated and involved.

I share this analogy with my patients in the hopes of impressing upon them the importance of relevant, early diagnosis.

YOUR PRECIOUS SIGHT

Chapter Key Points:

- The signs of retinal tear or detachment are seeing flashing lights or a sudden increase in the numbers of floaters, reduced peripheral (side) vision, and a curtain-like film/shadow over the visual field.
- When experiencing flashing lights or floaters, eyes need to be dilated, and the retina needs to be thoroughly evaluated.
- Retina tear or retinal detachment is an emergency. Without prompt treatment, it can lead to permanent vision loss.
- The risk factors for retinal tear or detachment include:
  - Moderate or extreme nearsightedness or high astigmatism.
  - Medications that constrict the pupil, like pilocarpine.
  - Certain systemic diseases, like diabetes and sickle cell disease.
  - History of eye injury.
  - History of eye surgery, like cataract or glaucoma.
  - History of retinal detachment in the other eye.
  - Family history of retinal detachment.

- History of eye diseases or thinness of retinal tissue with unknown reason.

Chapter 13

"I just want a second opinion."

The Stories about More than the Headaches, Double Vision, and Blurred Vision

---

"A stroke happens when blood supply to the brain is interrupted. Vision loss after stroke: Your vision depends on a healthy eye to receive information and a healthy brain to process that information. The nerves in the eye travel from the eye through the brain to the occipital cortex at the back of the brain, allowing you to see. Most strokes affect one side of the brain. Nerves from each eye travel together in the brain, so both eyes are affected."

~Stroke Foundation

MY PRACTICE PARTNER, Dr. Andrew R.

Lim, contributed to this case.

"My brother, Antonio, recommended seeing you," said Yolanda, a 42-year-old Hispanic woman. Her breathing was shallow and rapid as she took a white-knuckled grip on the arms of the exam chair. At first glance, I thought she was pregnant. Quickly, I checked her patient information sheet. She had marked that she was not pregnant, and she was under medication for diabetes. I was relieved that I hadn't asked how far along she was.

"I had a terrible headache, and I went to the emergency room two days ago. The doctor gave me some medication for migraines," she muttered with a frail voice.

I checked her ocular motility; there was no restriction on the eye muscle movement. Her physical condition concerned me, so I decided not to dilate her eyes. Nevertheless, I did take a digital retinal photograph, which revealed no evidence of diabetic retinopathy.

The confrontation visual field tests showed bilateral left homonymous hemianopia—she missed the entire left side of vision in both eyes—which indicated an insult on the occipital lobe of her brain.

YOUR PRECIOUS SIGHT

She was referred to her HMO emergency clinic instantly for a cerebral vascular accident (CVA) evaluation. With the referral letter, she was admitted to the hospital without further delay and diagnosed with a stroke.

Months later, she returned for a follow-up. She had lost all sight in one eye and retained partial vision in the other. She was on antidepressants and other medications for her health condition. I referred her to the Low Vision Clinic and encouraged her to be active and maintain good control of her diabetes.

Yolanda's incident had a tremendous impact on her brother, Antonio, who was overweight as well. He became an ardent cyclist and determined to be active and have a healthy lifestyle.

On a side note:

I have encountered a similar case. The patient was a slim, 35-year-old accountant with a chief complaint of progressive headaches for three months. She worked on the computer many hours a day as demanded by her profession. Her primary care physician diagnosed her as having migraines and recommended that she have an eye exam.

She had no other medical history. On pretesting, the autorefractor revealed mild farsightedness (hyperopia) in both eyes, which could be the cause of her headaches. However, her visual field test showed bilateral left homonymous hemianopia, similar to that of the previous patient.

She was referred to a neurologist as a walk-in on the same day. A few hours later, the neurologist called back. The neurological testing revealed that she had a brain tumor.

This patient was transferred to the care of her oncologist.

*"**Pseudotumorcerebri** literally means 'false brain tumor.' It is likely due to high pressure within the skull caused by the buildup or poor absorption of cerebrospinal fluid (CSF). If a diagnosis of pseudotumorcerebri is confirmed, close, repeated ophthalmologic exams are required to monitor any changes in vision."*

~NIH

YOUR PRECIOUS SIGHT

EMILY WAS ACCOMPANIED by her husband to have an exam. She had been our patient since high school. We had noticed her gradual weight gain in the last fifteen years, especially after having three kids. She was always sweet and joked about being overweight and her many diet failure stories.

"My neurologist recommended me to have an eye exam," she said as she slouched in the exam chair.

My ears perked up. "You've seen a neurologist?"

"Yeah, I suddenly started having double vision and terrible headaches, so my primary care physician referred me to a neurologist." She paused to catch her breath.

"What did he find out?"

"Nothing. He ran a CT scan on me and found *nothing* wrong." She sighed and hugged the big purse on her lap.

I went on to do a comprehensive eye exam. Her visual field was normal in both eyes. However, the cover test revealed intermittent esotropia (eyes turned inward) in both eyes, which was the cause of her double vision because her eyes were not aligned.

When I looked into her optic nerve head in a dilated fundus exam, the culprit of her trouble screamed aloud! Her optic nerve heads were edematous (swollen) with hemorrhaging (bleeding), both eyes. She had bilateral papilledema.

The digital retinal photography was printed out, along with a referral letter. She was instructed to take them to her neurologist *immediately*.

Two hours later, the neurologist called me. He stated that he reviewed the CT scan and still could not detect any abnormality; however, he admitted Emily to the hospital and ordered a spinal tap. The final diagnosis was that Emily had pseudotumorcerebri, false brain tumor.

She was on diuretic medications, and a spinal fluid shunt was put in place to reduce the pressure in her brain and drain the excess fluid. She was advised to lose weight because being overweight was believed to be one of the risk factors for pseudotumorcerebri.

Her vision returned to normal.

Seven years have passed since that double

vision and headache crisis. Her last eye exam showed no signs of permanent damage. Losing weight was still a challenge for her though.

For more information about pseudotumor-cerebri, please check out the References section at the back, under Chapter 13.

~ * ~

*"**Choroidal melanoma** is the most common primary intraocular (occurring inside the eye) tumor in adults. Because choroidal melanoma is intraocular and not usually visible, patients with this disease often do not recognize its presence until the tumor grows to a size that impairs vision by obstruction, retinal detachment, hemorrhage, or other complication. Pain is unusual, except with large tumors. Periodic retinal examination through a dilated pupil is the best means of early detection."*

~NEI

"I'M HERE FOR a second opinion. My coworker referred me." Joshua sat tall in the exam chair and offered me a warm smile. He bore a striking resemblance to a young Pierce Brosnan. His dark-brown tie, chestnut-and-purple plaid shirt, khaki pants, and tan oxfords were the very definition of casual business attire. His demeanor was both confident and charming.

I quickly looked over his patient information sheet. He was forty years old, a district manager for a high-end department store, on no medication, and he had worn contact lenses for twenty years. Other than the auto-refractor, which presented moderate nearsightedness and low astigmatism in both eyes, the pretests performed by my assistant were all within the normal range.

Why does he need a second opinion? LASIK surgery?

"Welcome to the office. What's the scoop?" The intriguing color of his eyes drew my attention. They were golden, and they almost shimmered as they reflected the overhead light.

"I've worn contact lenses for many years. A couple of years ago, my eye doctor fitted me with thirty-day disposable lenses. They were great because I traveled a lot. However, I started to have some problems about six months ago,"

YOUR PRECIOUS SIGHT

he said, frowning.

"What kind of problems?" I queried.

"The vision in my left eye was blurry. It bothered me. First, I thought my contact was dirty, so I changed to a new lens, but it didn't help. I went back to my eye doctor, and she switched me to one-day disposables. I still saw blurry in the left eye. I've been back to her a couple more times. Last time, she fitted me with the newest lenses on the market—at least that's what she told me. She said if that doesn't work she might fit me with multifocal, or one eye for distance and one eye for near, or something like that. She said everybody's eyes change around forty years old. I have an appointment with her tomorrow. But I wanted to get your opinion first."

I made some notes as he filled me in.

"Do you have the latest lenses with you?" I asked.

"Yeah, I just took them off." He handed me his contact lenses case. I inspected the lenses and recognized the brand.

"Your eye doctor was correct. These lenses are one of the newest on the market. Good stuff.

Let's go through the exam first, and then I'll let you know my findings and thoughts."

Joshua was attentive and alert through the exam. However, the best correctable vision was 20/20 on the right eye and 20/30 on the left eye.

"I need to dilate your eyes. Do you have a driver?"

"I can call my wife to pick me up," he responded.

Through the dilated fundus exam, I could see his right eye was intact, with no sign of tear or hole. In the left eye, there was a dome-shaped growth about seven optic discs in size, with some unusual pigmentation and vascular tortuosities.

I had my practice partner evaluate the retinal image; our concurrent diagnosis was choroidal melanoma, a kind of eye cancer.

Since Joshua had an excellent PPO insurance, we could refer him directly to an ocular oncologist at a reputable university eye center.

A week later, the ocular oncologist called me to confirm the diagnosis. He mentioned that they had found no distant metastasis, which was fantastic news. He also stated that he and

YOUR PRECIOUS SIGHT

his team would make all efforts to save Joshua's eye, which meant that they would do radiation therapy first, instead of enucleation (removal of the eye).

I couldn't even imagine him losing one of his stunning, golden eyes.

The ocular oncologist praised our timely diagnosis and appreciated our referral. Since Joshua's case was beyond our office's scope of practice, we transferred this case to the university eye center entirely.

My personal motto and advice to my patients and loved ones—including you, my dear readers—is "when in doubt, check it out."

Chapter Key Points:

- Most headaches are not a life-threatening medical situation. However, when you experience new symptoms that are unusual or more severe than typical, it's essential to be checked by your doctor.
- Pseudotumorcerebri (PTC), aka "idiopathic intracranial hypertension" or false brain tumor, is caused by the increase of fluid pressure in the brain.
- Prompt diagnosis and treatment of pseudotumorcerebri are critical because it may cause progressive or permanent vision loss.
- The vision problems associated with PTC develop slowly. They can be blurred vision or double vision. An eye exam may reveal that the optic nerve is swelling at the back of the eye, called papilledema.
- Choroidal melanoma is the primary eye cancer in adults. The symptoms of choroidal melanoma can be blurred vision, flashing lights, or floaters. It's rare to have pain, and many patients have no symptoms at all.
- According to the NEI, "The best way to detect an early choroidal melanoma is through

YOUR PRECIOUS SIGHT

a periodic comprehensive eye exam via a dilated pupil to evaluate the fundus (the back of the eye)."

Chapter 14

"I want to return my glasses."

The Stories of Diabetic Patients

*"**Diabetic eye disease** comprises a group of eye conditions that affect people with diabetes. These conditions include diabetic retinopathy, diabetic macular edema (DME), cataract, and glaucoma. The early stages of diabetic retinopathy usually have no symptoms. The disease often progresses unnoticed until it affects vision. Bleeding from abnormal retinal blood vessels can cause the appearance of 'floating spots.' Vision lost to diabetic retinopathy is sometimes irreversible. However, early detection and treatment can reduce the risk of blindness by 95 percent. Diabetic retinopathy and DME are detected during a comprehensive dilated eye exam."*

~NEI

YOUR PRECIOUS SIGHT

A DAY AFTER Christmas, the front office was filled with merriment. The lights cheerfully blinked on the artificial evergreen in the corner, and holiday music softly hummed in the background.

Suddenly, I heard a commotion. A voice bellowed through the office as a man bickered angrily with my lead assistant, Lisa. I was going through some mail from the other day and hoped the front office could resolve the conflict. Lisa had been with us for three years and was well trained. I had granted her some authority to manage challenging patients.

Through all the muffled noises, I got the impression that the patient wanted to return his glasses. We'd had a couple of occurrences in the past in which patients wanted to return a pair of glasses and demanded a full refund after use, often for absurd reasons. In one case, a woman wanted to return her deceased husband's glasses. "He doesn't need them anymore, wherever he is now," she stated. Another time, a patient insisted that she did not need her new pair of Versace glasses because her son's wedding was over and she had taken a good deal of photos with them on. "I want to return them and get my money back," she explained.

DR. EICHIN CHANG-LIM

I hoped this was not one of those obnoxious situations that would ruin my holiday spirit.

A few minutes later, Lisa walked in with a chart in her hand.

"Mr. Johns wants to return his glasses and get a refund," she said, shaking her head.

"What's the reason?" I inquired.

"He said the prescription is wrong. He can't see well with them any longer."

I reviewed the chart. I did the refraction and eye exam two weeks prior; he was happy with the prescription and signed off on the dispensing day. The medical history was all negative. The dilated fundus exam displayed some early signs of vascular changes, which were within the normal range for his age. The optic nerve head and fundus were within the normal range as well. Since the next patient was not ready to be seen, I told Lisa that I would do the recheck on Mr. Johns.

Mr. Johns, in his late fifties, sat stiffly in the exam chair, his arms crossed. He was wearing a navy blue sweatshirt printed with "This is What the World's Greatest GRANDPA Looks Like."

"Merry Christmas, Mr. Johns. Nice shirt."

YOUR PRECIOUS SIGHT

"Thanks," he replied coldly. I watched his jaw clench, and his lips tightened into a thin, straight line.

I endeavored to break the ice. "How many grandchildren do you have?"

"Three. And one on the way." His facial muscles relaxed. With that, I glided into his main complaint.

"The new pair of glasses worked fine until two days ago. Now everything looks blurry with them on." Hastily, he added, "I can read better without these glasses, as a matter of fact."

I rechecked his refraction, and he was right: the power of his prescription had changed dramatically in two weeks, from farsighted to nearsighted.

The two main reasons for a myopic shift — a change toward nearsightedness — are the development of a cataract or a change in the patient's blood sugar level. Since his cataract was fairly unchanged, I suspected that his blood sugar was the culprit.

One's blood sugar level can affect the shape of the crystalline lens—the natural lens behind the iris, about the size of an M&M—that can lead to fluctuating vision and require the alteration of an eyewear prescription. Most of the time, if a patient is known to have diabetes, we want to ensure that the patient's blood sugar level is stabilized before finalizing the eyewear prescription.

I shared with him my tentative diagnosis and filled out a referral form for his PCP. When I handed him the referral letter, I gave him a heads-up about the blood test and let him know I would like to follow up with him regarding his prescription. He was reluctant and insisted that he was perfectly healthy. Nevertheless, he agreed to defer the returning of glasses until after he visited his PCP and had a blood test.

Almost four months later, he returned for a follow-up. Indeed, the blood test revealed that he had diabetes, and it was now under control with the oral medication he received from his PCP. His PCP provided him with a wealth of information about the complications of diabetes and the importance of regular eye exams. He followed the protocol diligently.

He was one of the lucky ones to learn how to manage his diabetes before serious ocular manifestation transpired.

YOUR PRECIOUS SIGHT

~ * ~

"People with all types of diabetes (type 1, type 2, and gestational) are at risk for diabetic retinopathy. Risk increases the longer a person has diabetes. Between 40 and 45 percent of Americans diagnosed with diabetes have some stage of diabetic retinopathy, although only about half are aware of it. Women who develop or have diabetes during pregnancy may have rapid onset or worsening of diabetic retinopathy."

~NEI

THE FOLLOWING CASES were not unique. I lost count of how many similar cases I'd encountered in my years in the eye care profession. Mr. Lopez is an example.

He was in his forties, a truck driver who showed an expanded midsection but was not terribly overweight. He came in with his wife, a dark-haired, quiet lady. She gave me a nod and a smile as I came into the room. During the case history, Mr. Lopez was polite and stated that he considered himself fit and active when he was not on the road. He used nonprescription sunglasses during the daytime. This was his first eye exam because he had just received vision-care benefits through his new job.

"My eyes're playing tricks on me," he complained.

"What kind of tricks?" I asked him.

"I see okay most of the time. But at night I feel disoriented. I mean, the road signs seem to dance around sometimes."

He paused for a couple of seconds and then continued. "I just want to get a pair of glasses to see better after dark."

Since it was his first eye exam, we did the dilation and took the digital retinal fundus photo as baseline information. The central retina showed dot-and-flame hemorrhages with healthy macula. I turned the monitor toward him to present the images and explained the results to him. When I inquired about a recent physical exam and implied that he might have diabetes or other systemic involvements, he got agitated and defensive and insisted that he was perfectly healthy. Before I could provide further explanation, he jumped up and stormed out of the room. His face flushed, leaving his wife to pay the copay.

YOUR PRECIOUS SIGHT

"I am taking my prescription somewhere else. I will never come back here," he hollered upon exiting the front office.

A couple of weeks later, his wife and two kids came in to have eye exams with the newly acquired vision insurance benefits.

"My husband wanted to apologize to you for being abrupt the other day. I talked him into having a physical, and his fasting blood sugar level was 300 something. His PCP said he might have had diabetes for a while."

"No worries. I'm glad he got it checked," I replied to the sweet lady.

Mr. Lopez came in to have a digital fundus photo taken every six months from then on, which was covered by his insurance. Our office maintained close communication with his PCP to ensure his blood sugar was well managed. We routinely send a vision report to a diabetic patient's PCP after a comprehensive eye exam.

For patients like Mr. Lopez, our goal is to detect any early signs of change. If there was any indication of advancement in diabetic retinopathy, we would refer him to a retinal specialist to have laser photocoagulation or other treatment regimens. Ultimately, we want to preserve patients' eyesight for as long as possible.

Diabetes is one of the leading causes of blindness, not only in the USA but worldwide!

YOUR PRECIOUS SIGHT

Chapter Key Points:

The information is taken from the National Eye Institute (NEI), which is part of the federal government's National Institutes of Health (NIH). For further information, please check out the References section at the back, under Chapter 14.

- The early stages of diabetic retinopathy usually have no symptoms. The disease often progresses unnoticed until it affects vision. A regular comprehensive eye exam is the only way to detect and manage the disease in the early stages.
- Diabetic eye disease comprises a group of eye conditions that affect people with diabetes. These conditions include diabetic retinopathy, diabetic macular edema (DME), cataract, and glaucoma.
- All forms of diabetic eye disease have the potential to cause severe vision loss and blindness.
- Diabetic retinopathy involves changes to retinal blood vessels that can cause them to bleed or leak fluid, distorting vision.
- Diabetic retinopathy is the most common

cause of vision loss among people with diabetes and a leading cause of blindness among working-age adults.

- DME is a consequence of diabetic retinopathy that causes swelling in the area of the retina called the macula, which is responsible for the acute, central vision.
- Controlling diabetes—by taking medications as prescribed, staying physically active, and maintaining a healthy diet—can prevent or delay vision loss.
- Because diabetic retinopathy often goes unnoticed until vision loss occurs, people with diabetes should get a comprehensive dilated eye exam at least once a year.
- Early detection, timely treatment, and appropriate follow-up care of diabetic eye disease can protect against vision loss.
- Diabetic retinopathy can be treated with several therapies, used alone or in combination.
- NEI supports research to develop new therapies for diabetic retinopathy and to compare the effectiveness of existing therapies for different patient groups.

Chapter 15

"Am I getting old?"

The Stories of Needing Reader or Multifocal Lenses

---

*"**Presbyopia** is a common type of vision disorder that occurs as you age. It is often referred to as the aging eye condition. Presbyopia results in the inability to focus up close, a problem associated with refraction in the eye."*

~NEI

WHEN WE APPROACH the magic 40-year-old milestone mark, our body gently, yet cruelly, nudges us to remind us of the passing of time. Besides the midlife crisis, our eyes begin to cause us trouble.

I heard patients complaining:

"My arms are getting too short." (This was said more often in the case of farsighted patients or the ones used to have perfect vision.)

"I read better when I take my glasses off." (I heard this frequently from my nearsighted patients.)

"The writing on the medicine bottles is shrinking."

"I have to enlarge the font on my smartphone."

It's comforting to know that these changes are universal as we age, regardless of a person's social or economic status. There is a medical term for this condition in vision; it's called presbyopia. Keep in mind that it's not a disease; it's a natural part of the aging process.

"Am I getting old?" is a legitimate question, asked by almost everyone when I mentioned presbyopia.

My response is usually, "You're not getting older; you're getting wiser and better." I say that as a reminder to myself as well, because I have far surpassed the 40-year-old mark.

What happens is that the flexibility of our natural (crystalline) lens and of the muscle fibers around the lens diminishes with time, which affects the accommodative ability to see close-up. Accommodation is like taking close-up photos of objects; you need to dial in extra power to get the image of the objects captured through the camera lens in focus.

The solution is easy; we just need eyewear to compensate for the weakening accommodation. Nowadays, there are several options. Instead of just writing down a prescription, I spend extra time to explain the choices for the first-time wearers of multifocal lenses. Those options include:

- Two pairs of glasses—one for distance and one for near vision.
- Single vision lenses for reading, if a person has perfect distance vision.
- Multifocal lenses with line(s): bifocal or trifocal.
- Multifocal lenses with no line, known as progressive lenses.

No one solution is right for everyone. My advice is to be sure to ask the optician who fills your prescription about the pros and cons of each option; do not let them tell you what to get. Also, you need to communicate with the optician about your lifestyle, occupation, and needs.

If you find yourself a bit traumatized or depressed about the switch to multifocal lenses, or if you're suddenly in need of glasses for the first time, you're not alone.

The change can be overwhelming, but once you see clearly, both up-close and far away, it will be much easier to adjust to it.

~ * ~

Contact lens wearers face similar frustrations as they reach their forties, especially when it comes to close-up vision.

First of all, our eyes tend to get drier as we age, which makes wearing contact lenses less comfortable. Patients also encounter difficulty with seeing near with contact lenses that have served them well for years.

The options to help my contact lens patients overcome the near-vision challenges are:

Both single-vision contact lenses fitted for

distance and a pair of glasses to wear over contact lenses for near vision.

- Both single-vision contact lenses fitted for near vision and a pair of glasses to wear over contact lenses for distance.
- Monovision: single-vision contact lenses fitted on one eye for near vision and one eye for distant vision.
- Multifocal contact lenses for both eyes.
- Modified monovision: a single-vision lens on one eye and a multifocal lens on the other.

One-day disposable lenses are my preferred wearing modality, especially for dry-eye patients, because dirty lenses drastically reduce the wettability. Successful contact lens wearing takes a vast amount of time, with trial lens fittings, adjustments, follow-ups, and frequent communication required. Don't be frustrated if your eye doctor has to try different powers or various brands to find the best fit for you, especially for monovision and multifocal lens users.

Remember, contact lenses are not like a pair of shoes that you can slip on and forget about them. I encourage all of my contact lens patients to have a pair of glasses as a backup. I always prescribe monovision lens wearers a pair of glasses to wear over their contact lenses, so both eyes see equally clearly for distance, especially when driving at night.

For detailed information about bifocal or multifocal contact lenses, please check out the References section at the back under Chapter 15.

~ * ~

Refractive surgery is one of the means to correct presbyopia. I always candidly and deliberately communicate my point with patients that presbyopia is a progressive condition, continuing until around sixty-five years of age. Many people will have cataracts at that age, and cataract surgery is one of the procedures to correct refractive errors.

Why not wait until then?

If a patient does not want to wait until then and seriously contemplates the refractive surgery for presbyopia at an earlier age, I refer them to a reputable surgeon for evaluation and consultation. Nevertheless, I veer toward

YOUR PRECIOUS SIGHT

a conservative stance on this issue.

~ * ~

Let me share a couple of my favorite quotes about aging before leaving this chapter.

"You are never too old to set another goal or to dream a new dream."

~C. S. Lewis

"Know that you are the perfect age. Each year is special and precious, for you shall only live it once. Be comfortable with growing older."

~Louise Hay

Chapter Key Points:

- Presbyopia is an ocular condition defined as the gradual loss of the eye's ability to focus sharply on close-up objects.
- Presbyopia is not a disease; it is a part of the normal aging process.
- As we age, our eyes get drier. It can become a challenge to wear contact lenses comfortably.
- Evaluate your lifestyle and personal preferences. Communicate openly with your eye care professional to discover the best option to meet your vision needs. Many times, it requires trial and error to find the optimal solution to overcome vision changes due to presbyopia.

Chapter 16

"I cannot stop tearing. My eyes are on fire."

The Stories of Dry Eyes

***Dry eye** occurs when the quantity and/or quality of tears fails to keep the surface of the eye adequately lubricated. Experts estimate that dry eye affects millions of adults in the United States.*

~NEI

"WELCOME TO OUR office," I greeted Elma. She was a new patient in her early thirties, with lavender-tinged, platinum-blonde hair cut in a long bob.

"You're on my vision service plan. I found you online," she said in a matter-of-fact tone.

The skin around Elma's eyes was red and raw. Her tears welled up. "I hate that air puff test. It made me cry." She was referring to the noncontact tonometry, a test to measure the pressure inside a person's eye. I handed her the box of Kleenex. Her thick eyeliner and heavy mascara had smeared, giving her a hint of raccoon eyes.

"This Santa Ana wind makes me cry. My eyes are on fire, like someone smeared chili on my eyeballs." Elma dabbed her eyes. I was glad she shifted the blame to the weather instead of the air puff test.

"I'm a graphic designer in a marketing firm and have to work on the computer all the time. This is driving me crazy. I thought I had allergies, so I took Allegra."

"Did it work?" I asked. In the meantime, I made a mental note that she did not blow her nose. She had red eyes, but no red, runny nose.

She shrugged. "Not really."

I started going down the list of questions.

"Taking other medications?"

"Birth control pills and an antidepressant. Um, Prozac."

"Are you smoking?"

YOUR PRECIOUS SIGHT

"Yes. More lately, because of stress at work."

"Do you use contact lenses?" I didn't see contact lenses on her bloodshot brown eyes, but I asked anyway.

"Yes, colored lenses with no power. I had LASIK six years ago. I only wear them to change my eye color. But for the last few days I haven't been able to keep the lenses on."

At this point, I had a good idea of what she had. I went through the exams to confirm my diagnosis.

Elma had a touch of farsightedness. The slit lamp exam showed a faint circular line along the peripheral cornea of each eye, where the flap from her LASIK surgery had been. I had her close her eyes, and I gently dabbed them dry. Then I checked her tear break-up time (TBUT) using sodium fluorescein dye and the slit lamp. It was around seven seconds for each eye. (Normal TBUT is above ten seconds.) I pull down her lower lids; her tear prisms were much less than normal on both eyes. There were many other dry-eye tests to determine the origin of the problems, but I decided not to get too complicated. Based on her chief complaints and my findings, the diagnosis was dry eye. Her teary eyes were reflex tears triggered by the irritation from dry-eye syndrome.

Not all dry-eye patients experience the same signs and symptoms, which can include stinging, burning, itchiness, redness, fluctuating vision, irritation, grittiness, foreign body sensations, watery eyes, light sensitivity, contact lens intolerance, and eye fatigue, to name a few.

The culprits of dry eyes are numerous. Elma had assembled a great number of them to substantiate her problem, compounded with the unfavorable weather: smoking; taking medications like birth control pills, antihistamines, and antidepressants; working at the computer for prolonged hours; a history of laser eye surgery; wearing contact lenses; and applying eyeliner along the Meibomian glands—the oil glands along the eyelashes, responsible for the secretion and supply of the oil layer of the outer tear film.

Given that this was our first encounter, I genuinely wanted to establish a good relationship with her. I refrained from sounding like a nagging mother or a stern priest. I acknowledged her distress and let her know there were millions of Americans suffering from dry-eye syndrome every day; she was not alone.

I told her to stop taking the allergy pill, not to wear contact lenses for a while, and to avoid applying eyeliner inside the eyelash line. Last but not least, I advised her to stop smoking.

I gave her some samples of non-preservative single-dose artificial tears and prescribed a pair of computer glasses. I also reminded her to blink regularly and give her eyes a break every twenty minutes.

"Return for a follow-up in a week," I said as I walked her to the front office to make the appointment.

"By the way, I like your hair," I told her before transferring the chart to my assistant.

"Dry eye and Meibomian gland dysfunction are largely modern diseases, having recently increased in incidence, and it is an important public health problem. Although proper eyelid care will ensure the health of the ocular surface, its habit in general population has not previously been

reported."

~Motoko Kawashima, MD, PhD.

ONE WEEK LATER, Elma came in to pick up her computer glasses—dark-tortoiseshell, modified-cat-eye frames with antireflective and blue light blocking coating. She looked professional and chic at the same time. She was thrilled.

Her teary eyes problem had subsided. I noticed she had toned down her eye makeup a great deal compared to a week before.

It's time to talk to her about ocular hygiene and healthy tears!

When we shed tears of sorrow or joy, those tears are not just clear, water-like liquid. If you've ever tasted those tears that roll down your cheeks and land on your lips, they taste salty. It's because our tear fluid actually contains many chemical components to protect our eyes. I shared the following information with Elma and other patients using a helpful tear-film diagram.

The tear film on the surface of our eyes has three layers: the mucin layer—the inner layer to help the tears spread, stick to and nourish the underlying cornea; the water layer—the middle layer to lubricate the eye and wash out impurities; and the oil layer—the lipid-based outer layer that serves as a sealer to prevent the water layer from drying out.

The outermost oil layer was produced by the Meibomian glands, which align alongside our upper and lower eyelash lines. Meibomian glands, like other oil glands in our body, can become clogged, blocked, infected, and inflamed. When Meibomian glands become dysfunctional, the water layer evaporates quickly, the eyelids become red and crusty, and dry-eye disease and blepharitis develop.

Ocular hygiene maintains the health of the Meibomian glands by keeping them clean and open. These are the steps to clean them:

- Use warm compresses for five minutes
- Soak a clean piece of cloth in a baby shampoo diluted with warm water
- Gently rub the base of eyelashes with the cloth
- Rinse with warm water

In our office, we had a handout for patients to

take home, depicting the steps in detail. You can check the article, *Do-It-Yourself Eyelid Scrub for Itchy Eyes by Troy Bedinghaus, OD* in the References section at the back, under Chapter 16.

"Just as you need to brush your teeth daily for good dental hygiene, you need to scrub your eyelids daily to maintain healthy lids and tear film," I told Elma. I gave her some samples of fish oil, which is believed to be beneficial for our eyes, and commercial lid scrub before she left.

Three months later, Elma returned and requested contact lenses fitting. Since her teary problem from dry eyes had mostly resolved, she wanted opaque color contacts to change her eye color for fun. I recommended one-day disposables, and she accepted it without fuss.

Hooray! I'd gained her trust!

Now, she changed her brown eyes to blue when she didn't need to work long hours on the computer, and she always had fresh, brand-new lenses for optimal comfort.

~ * ~

YOUR PRECIOUS SIGHT

According to the 2012 Gallup poll, 26 million Americans suffer from dry eyes, and the number is expected to increase to 29 million by 2022. The prevalence of dry-eye disease is indisputable.

Current dry-eye treatments include artificial tears, Restasis, Xiidra, steroid eye drops, Lacrisert, punctal plugs, Meibomian gland expression, warm compresses, LipiFlow, Intense Pulsed Light, nutritional supplements, and home remedies for dry eyes. Our practice and co-management ophthalmologists recommended and performed all of the treatments based on the severity of a patient's dry-eye disease.

To understand more about what each treatment entails, please check out the References section at the back, under Chapter 16.

I need to mention one other mode of dry-eye treatment, which is autologous serum or autologous plasma eye drops. These are custom eye drops, made in a lab using a patient's own blood serum and plasma. Our practice and our co-management ophthalmologists shied away from prescribing this particular treatment due to its varying efficacy, high cost, and the additional hassle a patient incurs to get it. However, there have been some positive reports on the use of custom eye drops for dry-eye treatment.

For the sake of completeness in presenting dry-eye therapies, please visit the References section at the back, under Chapter 16.

YOUR PRECIOUS SIGHT

Chapter Key Points:

- An eye care professional who has examined your eyes and is familiar with your ocular and medical history is the best person to answer specific questions about your dry-eye symptoms.
- The signs and symptoms of dry-eye disease vary widely from individual to individual. They can include fluctuated vision, burning, stinging, watery eyes, irritation, itchiness, grittiness, redness, light sensitivity, foreign body sensation, contact lens intolerance, and fatigued eyes.
- The causes of dry-eye disease include the following: environmental factors (wind, smoke, or dry air), aging, hormonal variation, birth control pills, allergy, antihistamines or other systemic medications, prolonged digital device usage, contact lenses wearing, history of LASIK surgery, eye makeup misuse, Meibomian gland dysfunction, and cornea or eyelid diseases.
- The Meibomian glands along the upper and lower eyelids secrete oils onto the surface of the eye, preventing premature evaporation of the tear film.

- The use of heavy eye makeup can clog the Meibomian glands and cause Meibomian gland dysfunction, which leads to or worsens dry-eye disease and blepharitis.
- Eyelid hygiene is clinically relevant, no matter what stage of the dry-eye condition a person is experiencing.
- Multiple dry-eye treatments can be used, based on the severity of the problem and a patient's ocular and medical history. Treatment options may be artificial tears, Restasis, Xiidra, steroid eye drops, Lacrisert, punctal plugs, Meibomian gland expression, warm compresses, LipiFlow, Intense Pulsed Light, nutritional supplements, and home remedies.

Chapter 17

"Can you prescribe more of this drop for my mom?"

The Stories of Open-Angle Glaucoma (Silent Thief of Sight) and Acute Angle-Closure Glaucoma

---

"Glaucoma is a group of diseases that damage the eye's optic nerve and can result in vision loss and blindness. However, with early detection and treatment, you can often protect your eyes against serious vision loss."

~NEI

MRS. MARIA VALEDEZ smiled as she sat quietly in the exam chair. She gazed over at the young lady sitting in the armchair in the corner as I got ready to commence the case history. Per a prearranged agreement, I assumed, the daughter would do all the talking for Mrs. Valedez.

"My mother wants you to prescribe her a drop for her itchy eyes."

Then the daughter reached into her purse and fumbled around. After about twenty seconds of digging, she wrinkled her nose, furrowed her brows, and upended her handbag onto the empty chair next to her. A lipstick rolled over the edge of the chair, clattered to the floor, and kept rolling. Finally, she picked up a small bottle from among the chewing gum, keys, and other personal belongings.

"This one," the daughter said as she handed me the small bottle with a yellow cap. "She liked this one for her itchy eyes."

"Where did she get these drops?" My stomach reeled. I couldn't help but raise my voice.

After a brief conversation between the two of them, the daughter said, "She thinks she got it in Texas." She paused for a second and added, "My mother used to live with my brother in Texas. Then she went back to Colombia for two years. Now, she's living with me."

YOUR PRECIOUS SIGHT

Even though some of the letters on the bottle had been rubbed off, I could tell without ambiguity that this yellow-capped ophthalmic drop was Timoptic, a glaucoma medication. It is not intended for itching eyes! It's always a nightmare for physicians and pharmacists when a patient messes up the medication.

Instead of wasting time scrutinizing the source of the drops or making remarks that they might find insulting, I dove into the examination.

Why was she given this med? I wondered.

The comprehensive exam confirmed my suspicion; it revealed that her optic nerve head had a 0.7 cup-to-disc (C/D) ratio. (The cup is a pit with no nerve fibers. The disc is the pink rim containing the nerve fibers.) A normal C/D is around 0.3. The increase C/D ratio indicated the diminishing of nerve fibers. Her intraocular pressure (IOP) measured in the high 20s in each eye. A normal IOP is around 12-22 mmHg. During the perimetry test (visual field test), she was unable to keep her eyes open to complete the exam. It was late in the afternoon; she must have been exhausted.

My assistant brought both mother and

daughter back into the exam room. I communicated the findings and diagnosis with the daughter, who translated them to her mother sentence by sentence.

"Your mother has an eye disease called chronic open-angle glaucoma. It can cause blindness if untreated. Someone before must have diagnosed her with this disease. Her eye drops are the prescription used to treat it." Then I went through the nature of chronic open-angle glaucoma using an eye model. My script went like this:

"Our eye is like a ball filled with fluid. There is a system continuously producing the fluid and a system continuously draining the fluid. If the production is too fast or drainage is too slow or blocked, the pressure in the eye builds up and pushes on the optic nerve, and the nerves slowly die. If untreated, the side vision slowly shrinks in, and the person becomes blind." I paused to let the daughter translate, and then I picked up the bottle with the yellow cap again. "These drops would lower the pressure in your mother's eyes."

I had the front office schedule Mrs. Valedez to return the next morning to recheck the IOP and redo the visual field test. According to clinical reports, the IOP has diurnal fluctuation; it is highest in the morning.

Mrs. Valedez did not show up the next day. I had my Spanish-speaking assistant call her and reschedule. This call and no-show scenario went on for a week.

Finally, my office manager, who was also bilingual, called her and stated that if she did not receive treatment for her glaucoma, she would go blind. She even went the extra mile to tell Mrs. Valedez that *blindness* meant the light would be turned dark on her; she would see nothing, as if someone had blindfolded her.

One morning, Mrs. Valedez returned. Her IOP was in the low 30s. I referred her to a glaucoma specialist for surgical consultation and treatment.

Both my practice partner and I are glaucoma licensed; we are capable of diagnosing and treating glaucoma therapeutically. However, we sometimes refer patients—such as those who are noncompliant, have difficulty in handling drops, or for whom drops alone do not sufficiently control the IOP—out to glaucoma specialists. There are various laser and surgical procedures to lower IOP by enhancing the drainage system. The glaucoma specialist will monitor the patient's IOP to determine whether further therapy, like drops, or a procedure is needed.

Glaucoma can develop even the IOP is within the normal range. This form of glaucoma is called low-tension or normal-tension glaucoma. It is a type of open-angle glaucoma.

Patient management is crucial in treating glaucoma. The goal is to help the patient maintain the eyesight by all means. No one wants to be the last eye doctor the patient sees before he or she goes blind.

~ * ~

*"In **angle-closure glaucoma**, the fluid at the front of the eye cannot drain through the angle and leave the eye. The angle gets blocked by part of the iris. People with this type of glaucoma may have a sudden increase in eye pressure. Symptoms include severe pain and nausea, as well as redness of the eye and blurred vision. If you have these*

symptoms, you need to seek treatment immediately."

~NEI

"**DR. CHANG-LIM**, someone in the front office wants to see you," one of my assistants said.

"Something serious? Where's the patient's chart?"

"Nothing like that. She just wants to say hello."

Mrs. Dodson's eyes twinkled, and a warm, genuine smile lit up her face as I approached the front desk.

"Dr. Chang-Lim, I just wanted to stop by to thank you. The ER doctor said you saved my eyesight." In a quick motion, she reached out and wrapped me in a bear hug. Then she removed a box of See's Candies from her oversized canvas tote bag. "Here. For you!"

I sensed all eyes in the reception and dispensing areas on us. I could feel I was blushing.

I invited Mrs. Dodson to join me in the exam room so we could be in private for a minute.

DR. EICHIN CHANG-LIM

This is how the story of "saving Mrs. Dodson's eyesight" unfolded:

About one month prior, she was in our office for a yearly exam. With her diabetes, I should have dilated her pupils for a thorough fundus exam. However, I was reluctant to do so, because the drainage angle—the junction formed by the iris and cornea—in both of her eyes was narrow. I was afraid dilation would close the angle and block the drainage completely. In addition, it's an excellent strategy to perform a laser iridotomy prophylactically, which creates a hole in the outer edge of the iris to form a drainage channel in case the narrow angle closed for any reason. I decided to refer her out to a glaucoma specialist, though her IOPs were in the normal range then.

With her kind of insurance, she had to see her primary care physician (PCP) before seeing a specialist. Her PCP would submit the paperwork and make a request to her insurance company to obtain an authorization to see the specialist within her network.

As I handed her the referral letter, I went through the major symptoms of acute angle-closure glaucoma, which include headache, blurred vision, red eyes, eye pain, halos around lights, mid-dilated pupil, nausea, abdominal pain, and vomiting. The symptoms can mimic stomach flu or food poisoning in some cases.

"Remember, the acute angle closure is a real emergency. If you experience something like what I just told you, you need to be seen right away. You can go blind if you don't lower the pressure in your eyes quickly." I knew those words must sound grave to her ears. She made an appointment with her PCP right away. However, the lapse time for her PCP's appointment was two weeks.

One week after I saw her, her kids treated her to Cirque de Soleil for her sixtieth birthday. In the midst of the acclaimed performance, she developed a headache and some of the symptoms I'd told her about.

Her internal alarm system went off!

"I had my kids take me to the emergency room. There were many people there. I just yelled, 'Help me! I have angle-closure glaucoma. I'm going blind!' A nurse came, and I handed her your referral letter," Mrs. Dodson said, recalling the entire event with great animation. Fortunately, she caught the ER staff's attention promptly. Whatever they did, they managed to lower her eye pressure in a timely manner, and she received the laser treatment the next morning.

"Okay, let me take a look at your eyes," I said, helping her get settled behind the slit lamp after she told me about the laser treatment. Indeed, there was a nice, tiny hole on the periphery of both brown irises. "Looks great, Mrs. Dodson," I said with a smile.

"You saved my eyesight," she said again.

"I believe someone up there is watching over you." I meant it.

Perhaps I did a good job in frightening her.

The following is a list of things you should know about glaucoma, issued by NEI.

- More than 2.7 million Americans over age 40 have glaucoma.
- Anyone can develop glaucoma. The following groups are at higher risk of glaucoma:

YOUR PRECIOUS SIGHT

- – African Americans over age 40, people over age 60 (especially Mexican Americans),
  – And people with a family history of glaucoma.
- Getting a *comprehensive dilated eye exam* is the *only* way to catch glaucoma early.
- Don't wait for symptoms.
- Glaucoma damages the eye's optic nerve.
- Once glaucoma damages your optic nerve, lost vision *cannot* be restored.
- Eye pressure is a major risk factor for glaucoma.
- The only clinically proven treatment for glaucoma is to lower eye pressure.
- A new drug-delivery system is currently being tested.
- Studies in the laboratory and with patients are making key discoveries and giving new hope.

I am also including a link to "Facts About Glaucoma." Even though there are some redundancies in the information, it's worth reviewing multiple times, because glaucoma is one of the diseases deserving of attention. Please check out the References section at the back, under Chapter 17.

~ * ~

Last but not least . . .

Eye drops that contain steroids for treating ocular inflammation, and eye cream containing steroids for treating allergies and periorbital skin rash can induce IOP elevation. If using these, careful monitoring of the IOP by an eye care professional is mandatory.

Chapter Key Points:

- The two major kinds of glaucoma are chronic open-angle glaucoma and acute angle-closure glaucoma.
- There is a nickname for open-angle glaucoma, which is the "silent thief of sight." Because of its slow progress, one is rarely aware of any symptoms of this disease until it is in its late stage, when most of the irreversible damage to the optic nerve has been done. The only way to detect open-angle glaucoma early is by having a comprehensive eye exam on a regular basis.
- Acute angle-closure glaucoma is a real medical emergency. The draining system of the eye shuts down abruptly, and IOP elevates rapidly, which can damage the optic nerve head in a short time and cause permanent vision loss.
- "Glaucoma can develop without increased eye pressure. This form of glaucoma is called low-tension or normal-tension glaucoma. It is a type of open-angle glaucoma." ~NEI
- When the optic nerves die due to the increase in IOP, the cup-to-disc ratio increases

(the healthy nerves fibers diminish), the visual field constricts, and the peripheral vision reduces, becoming tunnel vision.
- The treatments for glaucoma aim at reduction in the fluid production and enhancement of fluid drainage. At times, a combination of therapeutical and surgical approaches is necessary to control the IOP to intervene in the optic nerve damage to prevent further vision loss.
- Be cautious that topical corticosteroids (drops, ointment, gel) on the eyes, eyelids, or skin around the eyes can raise IOP and lead to glaucoma.

Chapter 18

"It was a dark and stormy night..."

The Stories of Flashes of Light and Floaters

---

*"Most of the eye's interior is filled with vitreous, a gel-like substance that helps the eye maintain a round shape. There are millions of fine fibers intertwined within the vitreous that are attached to the surface of the retina, the eye's light-sensitive tissue. As we age, the vitreous slowly shrinks, and these fine fibers pull on the retinal surface. Usually the fibers break, allowing the vitreous to separate and shrink from the retina. This is a **vitreous detachment**."*

~NEI

I WAS ON my way to work when my cell phone rang. I let it go to voicemail and listened to the message once I got to the office.

"You need to see him this morning. You know, the man can act like a baby."

Lynda is my good friend; her husband, Ray, is my distant cousin. Ray is a freelance web developer, fifty-two years old at the time. Based on Lynda's message, Ray had experienced something "weird and frightening" in one of his eyes during the night. I called her right back.

"Bring him in right away. It sounds like I need to dilate his eyes. You'll need to drive him," I told her.

Lynda and Ray were already in the exam room when I finished with my first patient. I hugged them both.

"Tell me what happen…" I looked at Ray, expecting him to whimper like a baby, as Lynda had mentioned on the phone.

"It was a dark and stormy night . . ." Ray replied.

"Okay, Snoopy," I said, rummaging in my head for something equally witty to say to him. Lynda laughed in the corner. Then Ray stopped smiling, and a shadow crossed his face.

"I was working on my computer after midnight. I noticed small streaks of blue light in a

YOUR PRECIOUS SIGHT

red flash." Ray pointed to his right eye, with a little wink to confirm that it was the stormy one.

"Then it happened again about forty-five minutes later. The first time, I thought I was imagining it. The second time, I knew it was for real. It happened again about an hour later. It was so intense. After the third time, I was spooked. So I went to bed and hoped it would go away." He paused a beat and then continued. "This morning, as I got out of the bed, I saw that damn bright flashing light again. So I told Lynda, and she called you."

I quickly checked his IOP and anterior chamber to ensure the angles were open, with no signs of infection or inflammation. I dilated his eyes. There was no tear or hole on his central and peripheral fundus in either eye.

"Good news. You do not have retinal detachment. You have posterior vitreous detachment," I announced to Ray.

"What the heck is that?"

"Okay, Snoopy, let me explain. Our eyes are filled with vitreous, a gel-like substance. You can think of it as Jello. When we get older, the Jello liquefies and pulls away from the retina. The retina is the inner lining of our eyeballs and has millions of nerve endings within it. When the vitreous pulls away from the retina and stimulates the nerve endings, you see the bright flashing lights."

I assured him that the lightning in the stormy night would slowly subside as the liquefied Jello settled down. And it did calm down. A couple of months later, he updated his glasses prescription and was content.

However, something transpired again two years later.

"Lately, I've noticed my right-eye vision is not as sharp as before," he said when he came in to see me. "For the last two days, things have looked funny. When I cover my left eye, a straight line will look wavy with my right eye." Ray tilted his head and frowned at me.

With dilation and digital retinal photography, the diagnosis was that Ray had a macular pucker, which was a common result of the vitreous detachment. I shared some information from the National Eye Institute (NEI) with him.

"A macular pucker is scar tissue that has formed on the eye's macula, located in the center of the light-sensitive tissue called the retina. The macula provides the sharp, central vision we need for reading,

driving, and seeing fine detail. A macular pucker can cause blurred and distorted central vision. Macular pucker is also known as epiretinal membrane, preretinal membrane, cellophane maculopathy, retina wrinkle, surface wrinkling retinopathy, premacular fibrosis, and internal limiting membrane disease."

The best correctable vision in his right eye at the time was 20/60, which troubled him, and the distorted central vision interfered with his job. I referred him to a vitreoretinal specialist. After the consultation, and understanding the benefits and risks of the surgery, Ray consented to undergo the surgery, called vitrectomy. The procedure would peel and remove the thickened membrane and detach the tractional fibers, preventing a retinal tear.

Please remember, we are talking about operating on a *tiny* spot on the back of a human eyeball that is about two-thirds the size of a ping-pong ball!

The surgery was successful. The central distortion gradually went away.

Then, something changed again!

Seven months later, Ray's right-eye vision dropped to 20/60 once more. The decreased vision was due to the formation of cataracts, one of the side effects of vitrectomy the surgeon had forewarned him about.

The cataract surgery was a piece of cake compared to vitrectomy.

Three years later, his vision in his right eye was 20/20, which was remarkable and better than the eye surgeon had anticipated.

Indeed, it was incredible to achieve 20/20 vision after the series of events he'd experienced: posterior vitreous detachment, macular pucker, vitrectomy, and cataract surgery.

Hooray for the advance of modern medicine!

~ * ~

*"**Floaters** occur when the vitreous, a gel-like substance that fills about 80 percent of the eye and helps it maintain a round shape, slowly shrinks. As the vitreous shrinks, it becomes somewhat stringy, and the strands can cast tiny shadows on the retina. These are floaters. In most cases, floaters are part of the natural aging process and simply an annoyance. A sudden increase in floaters, possibly accompanied by light flashes or peripheral*

YOUR PRECIOUS SIGHT

(side) vision loss, could indicate a retinal detachment. A retinal detachment occurs when any part of the retina, the eye's light-sensitive tissue, is lifted or pulled from its normal position at the back wall of the eye."

~NEI

"I HATE THOSE little dots and lines floating in my eyes. They drive me crazy! So many times, I thought there was a bug flying over my face." As her husband's vision recovered, Lynda complained about the annoyance of floaters in both of her eyes.

Her complaint warranted some concern. She was -5 diopters of nearsightedness before LASIK sixteen years before. I had dilated her eyes several times since then. In fact, I had dilated her six weeks earlier and found no tears or holes at her peripheral or central fundus. Those little patches of lattice degeneration (thinning of the peripheral retina) on both eyes had revealed no changes all these years.

"Many people have floaters. I have them as well," I told her, forcing myself to hold back saying, *just live with it.*

While I was entering the information into the computer and contemplating whether I should dilate her again, Lynda picked up a copy of *People* magazine to fan herself with.

"Do you think menopause has anything to do with the increase of floaters?" she blurted, fanning even more vigorously.

"Oh, yeah. Trust me, menopause can do a lot to a person," Ray said, waggling his eyebrows in the corner.

I shot him a glare, and he promptly dropped his gaze back down to his iPad.

"Hey, be nice," Lynda grumbled.

Increase of floaters . . . Those words registered in my ears and hung in my head for a second.

That is not something to be ignored.

I grabbed the bottle and instilled the dilating agents in her eyes. Her pupils were widely dilated thirty minutes later.

With my binocular indirect ophthalmoscope (BIO) headset on and holding a 20 diopter lens, *I saw it.*

A chill ran down my spine.

OMG! I silently cried out.

YOUR PRECIOUS SIGHT

There was a retina tear at the 2 o'clock position on her left eye! She was referred to the retinal specialist immediately. The retinal specialist not only used the laser to seal the tear but also to strengthen the other weakening areas on both eyes, just as a precaution.

I could not begin to envision what might have happened if I had just brushed her off and assumed her complaints were due to the stress from her hormonal variations.

For the longest time, when I looked back on that day, I was haunted by guilt and shame. I'd considered my good friend a hypochondriac at what was, in reality, a perilous moment.

There is no absolute way to predict when a retinal tear might befall a person. The well-recognized risk factors are aging, a high degree of nearsightedness or astigmatism, thinning of the peripheral retina, family history of retinal tears or detachment, history of eye injury or eye surgery, and some systemic diseases, like diabetes. Moreover, a person may develop a retinal tear or detachment without any of the risk factors.

A regular comprehensive eye exam is the way to detect an asymptomatic tear or lattice degeneration (thinning of the retina) and manage the condition accordingly.

Early detection and treatment of a retinal tear/hole can prevent a full-blown retinal detachment. A retinal tear/hole is much easier to treat and less involved than a retinal detachment.

Chapter Key Points:

- Posterior vitreous detachment (PVD) is a natural occurrence with aging.
- The symptoms of PVD can include floaters and/or flashes. These symptoms tend to subside within several weeks. Some people may have PVD with no obvious symptoms at all.
- Most of the time, PVD is not a sight-threatening event; however, it can affect vision permanently if it involves retinal detachment, the formation of an epiretinal membrane (macular pucker), or macular hole.
- It's essential to get a professional diagnosis via a comprehensive dilated eye exam to confirm that flashing lights and floaters aren't related to a retinal tear, retinal detachment, or something even more serious.
- Retinal detachment or macular pucker can occur months or even years after the PVD.
- A sudden increase in the number of floaters can indicate changes in the retina. A prompt professional evaluation is needed.

Chapter 19

"Am I going blind? Should I take vitamins for my eyes?"

The Stories of Age-Related Macular Degeneration (AMD)

---

*"**AMD** is a common eye condition and a leading cause of vision loss among people age 50 and older. It causes damage to the macula, a small spot near the center of the retina and the part of the eye needed for sharp, central vision, which lets us see objects that are straight ahead. The early and intermediate stages of AMD usually start without symptoms. Only a comprehensive dilated eye exam can detect AMD."*

~NEI

I TURNED THE monitor of the Topcom retinal

camera toward Mr. Wong, a 67-year-old gentleman. We had been following-up on the drusen on his fundus for the last seven years. Drusen are yellow fatty-protein deposits under the retina, which increase a person's risk of developing AMD. The number of drusen on Mr. Wong's eyes had increased in the last two years, and some of them were clustered. Nevertheless, his central vision had been 20/20 in each eye since his cataract surgery with IOL (intraocular lenses) four years before.

"I'd like to refer you to a retinal specialist to have a good checkup and an OCT. Drusen can turn into macular degeneration in some cases," I said, choosing my words with discretion. It might have been overkill to refer someone to a retinal specialist at this stage; however, playing it safe has always been my strategy. An optical coherence tomography (OCT) is an imaging test, superior to a digital fundus camera, used to monitor a person's retinal changes over time.

Mr. Wong rested his elbow on the camera table and supported his chin with his big palm. He stared right into my eyes. "Am I going blind?"

"No, you're not. Even if you had advanced AMD, it would affect your central vision only. The light would not turn dark on you. You would still have peripheral vision, unless there were some other complications," I said, straightforward and upbeat. I did not want to mention the definition of "legally blind" at this time. We would talk about it later if it came down to it.

"I've listened to what you've said. I mean, I stopped smoking, eat better, wear sunglasses outdoors, and take vitamins," he said.

"You're doing all the right things!"

"Is there any treatment for macular degeneration?" Mr. Wong was thinking ahead.

"There have been many promising breakthroughs in recent years—things like ocular injections and laser surgery to restore vision. Also, there is ongoing research and development in this area. The future is hopeful. Anyway, I don't want you to lose sleep thinking you have it now." I reassured him and handed him the referral to a trusted retinal specialist.

In addition, I gave him the take-home Amsler grid, a simple test for monitoring macular changes at home, and explained how to use it correctly.

YOUR PRECIOUS SIGHT

Amsler Chart to Test Your Sight:

The Amsler grid is used to check whether lines look wavy or distorted and whether areas of the visual field are missing.

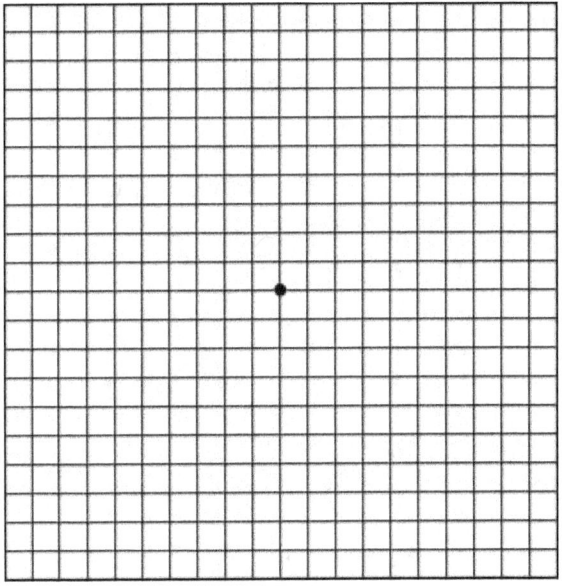

Tape this page at eye level where light is consistent and without glare.

Put on your reading glasses and cover one eye.

Fix your gaze on the center black dot.

Keeping your gaze fixed, try to see if any lines are distorted or missing.

Mark the defect on the chart.

TEST EACH EYE SEPARATELY.

If the distortion is new or has worsened, arrange to see your eye doctor at once.

Always keep the Amsler chart the same distance from your eyes each time you test.

This chart is provided by the American Macular Degeneration Foundation. Please check the References section at the back for the download link, under Chapter 19.

~ * ~

"There is no known treatment that can prevent the early stages of AMD. However, the AREDS formulations may delay progression of advanced AMD and help you keep your vision longer if you have intermediate AMD, or advanced AMD in one eye. The participants in the first AREDS trial have now been followed for 10 years, and the benefits

YOUR PRECIOUS SIGHT

of the AREDS formulation have persisted over this time."

~ NEI

I WAS AT an eye care symposium to earn part of the fifty hours of continuing education (CE) credits I'm required to accumulate every two years in order to renew my professional license. I always enjoy this particular symposium, not only because it consistently invites not-so-boring speakers and is a good complement to Vision Expo, but also because it provides the audience a good lunch, especially the satisfying dessert.

It was the last lecture before lunch. The slide on the multiple screens showed a woman standing in a supermarket aisle, her head tilted, her eyebrows furrowed. The shelves displayed rows and rows of ocular vitamins. Some had the image of a human eye; others had "AREDS2" printed on them. Obviously, she was frustrated and confused, being faced with copious choices. I could easily envisage her as one of my patients.

What in the world is AREDS all about?

AREDS stands for the Age-Related Eye Disease

Study. In 2001, a group of researchers based at the NIH's National Eye Institute (NEI) reported a formulation of nutritional supplements that could reduce the risk of developing age-related macular degeneration (AMD). This formula consisted of vitamin C, vitamin E, beta-carotene, zinc, and copper.

AREDS2 was the second study that began in 2006. In this study, lutein, zeaxanthin, and omega-3 fatty acids were added; beta-carotene was removed; and the dose of zinc was lowered. To understand the detailed report of AREDS, I strongly encourage you to check out the article link I shared in the References section at the back of this book.

Allow me to share with you the key question and answer from this article.

"What formulation should I take?" The answer from NEI is as follows:

Consult your doctor or eye care professional about which supplement, if any, is right for you. The ingredients based on AREDS and AREDS2 research are:

500 milligrams (mg) of vitaminC

400 international units of vitamin E

YOUR PRECIOUS SIGHT

80 mg zinc as zincoxide

2 mg copper as cupricoxide

10 mg lutein and 2 mg zeaxanthin

"Do you take vitamins?" my patients often ask when I mention vitamins for eyes.

"Of course!" is my answer.

According to the NEI, "The AREDS formulation is not a substitute for a multivitamin. In the AREDS trial, two-thirds of the study participants took multivitamins along with the AREDS formulation. In AREDS2, almost nine of ten participants took multivitamins."

However, I urge all of my patients to consult their primary physicians before rushing out to get any kind of vitamins. It's also essential to inform the pharmacist regarding all the prescribed medications, OTC drugs, vitamins, or even recreational drugs you are taking.

Too much of a good thing can be detrimental!

~ * ~

The risk factors for age-related macular degeneration

are aging, smoking, family history of AMD, UV light, blue light from digital devices, being overweight, and hypertension (high blood pressure).

AMD is identified by three different stages: early, intermediate, and advanced/late AMD. You may have heard the terms Dry AMD and Wet AMD. Wet AMD refers to the advanced stage when the fragile and abnormal blood vessels (neovascular) develop under the retina and lead to fluid leaking, bleeding, scarring, and vision loss.

Please check out the References section at the back under Chapter 19, for the link where you can learn the facts and stages of age-related macular degeneration.

Chapter Key Points:

- The macula is a small spot on the retina responsible for the most acute and central vision. Any insult on the macula will affect the vision greatly.
- Age-related macular degeneration (AMD) is a slow, progressive disease. The early and intermediate stages of AMD usually start without symptoms. Only a comprehensive dilated eye exam can detect AMD.
- AMD is a common eye condition and a leading cause of vision loss among people age fifty and older.
- Drusen are fatty deposits that accumulate in the retina. As a part of the normal aging process, having a few drusen is not uncommon. It's not a definite indication of AMD. However, having drusen is a risk factor for developing AMD and can be an early sign of macular degeneration, which needs to be monitored regularly.
- The risk of advanced AMD and vision loss is strongly related to the number, characteristics, and size of drusen.

- When drusen get larger and progress to the advanced stage, bleeding occurs, the macular scars, and central vision decreases.
- Taking AREDS2 formulation is reported to significantly slow the progress of drusen, delay the advance of AMD, and preserve the central vision longer.
- The treatments for advanced neovascular AMD, which occurs in the last stage as the new and abnormal blood vessels develop and lead to bleeding and scarring, are injections, photodynamic therapy, and laser surgery. There are ongoing researches and developments in this area.
- The risk factors for age-related macular degeneration are aging, smoking, family history of AMD, UV light, blue light from digital devices, being overweight, and hypertension (high blood pressure).

Chapter 20

"Everything appears as though looking through a dirty window and lights are glary."

The Stories about Cataracts and Cataract Surgeries

---

*"A **cataract** is a clouding of the lens in the eye that affects vision. Most cataracts are related to aging."*

~NEI

"YOUR CATARACT IS more jelly-like and sticky than other cataracts I have removed." In a semiconscious state, I believe that's what my surgeon, Dr. Hartman, said. I was on the operating table undergoing cataract surgery.

I was not even fifty years old, and I'd already undergone cataract surgery on my right eye!

I eat healthy, have never been overweight, and wear my sunglasses and hat diligently when I play golf. Most of my patients who have had a cataract are much older than I am. It certainly bugged me. The only thing I could think of was that I had taken cholesterol medication, Pravachol, for about twenty years, though no conclusive clinical data supports the assertion that cataracts are one of the side effects of this medication. My cholesterol levels had been over 300 mg/dL since college, which was presumably due to heredity.

The human lens, locating right behind the pupil, is about the size of an M&M candy. The lens accommodates and focuses for the eye, functioning just as a lens would do for a camera. With cataracts, the normally clear lens becomes cloudy or discolored. Most cataracts are age-related and progress slowly.

Before I signed the consent form for the cataract surgery, I'd reviewed the signs and symptoms of cataract, which I had explained to my patients for years based on what I read in textbooks. To actually *experience* it was something else!

YOUR PRECIOUS SIGHT

At first, I noticed that the glare of oncoming headlights disoriented me when driving at night. Then, everything seemed hazy, like looking through a dirty window. My prescription glasses shifted toward myopia (nearsightedness) way faster than normal. A slit lamp exam by my fellow optometrist confirmed the diagnosis of cataract.

Once the diagnosis was made, the next step was to determine *when* to have the cataract removed. If my patient was an active driver, I referred them to the surgeon when the best correctable vision was worse than 20/40, because 20/40 is considered the minimum vision for safe driving. However, 20/40 vision is not a cut-and-dried criterion. If a patient expressed frustration about performing daily activities, or if their job demanded a clearer vision, I did not hesitate to refer them to the surgeon right away.

I did not delay the cataract surgery since clear vision is a definite must for me to perform my daily work. In addition, I had referred patients to this surgeon and had seen the outstanding outcomes; I had all the confidence in him. There was no fear in me when I was wheeled into the operating room that day.

Cataract surgery is performed to remove the cloudy, discolored natural lens and replace it with a clear, plastic, artificial lens called an intraocular lens (IOL.) It's a relatively safe procedure, and the success rate is high. Nevertheless, it is a surgical procedure. Following the doctor's instructions before and after the operation is paramount in order to avoid any potential risks.

On a side note, I had cataract surgery on my left eye two years later. Then I had a quick laser procedure to clear the posterior capsule opacification (PCO), a filmy deposit on the posterior capsule, a couple of years after the second cataract surgery.

The capsule is the thin, clear membrane covering the natural lens. Most of the capsule is left in place during cataract surgery to help hold the inserted intraocular lens. Posterior capsule opacification causes blurred vision due to the deposits of scar tissue or cells formed behind the IOL. PCO is treated by a quick, low-risk, in-office laser procedure.

~ * ~

"Cataract is detected through a comprehensive

YOUR PRECIOUS SIGHT

eye exam. The symptoms of early cataract may be improved with new eyeglasses, brighter lighting, anti-glare sunglasses, or magnifying lenses. If these measures do not help, surgery is the only effective treatment. Surgery involves removing the cloudy lens and replacing it with an artificial lens."

~NEI

MY DEAR AUTHOR friend Bob sent me a note two days after his first cataract surgery. He was absolutely exhilarated. He was not my patient, but he wanted to share the excitement with me. He reported that his distance vision was much better than what it had been long before he had any evidence of a cataract, and he was able to read a book comfortably that morning without his glasses.

Then he wrote, "So the point of this is twofold. First, it is one of the few things in life that appears to be a fix. Not just a management issue, like with pain or diabetes or such. Second, I did not fully understand how much my vision would improve. I thought it would be that they took the cloud out, but the preexisting refraction problems would be largely unchanged. After forty-eight hours, I am impressed and happy. I knew it should be better. But it was MUCH better. For once in life, the good news was better than just good."

He had the second eye operated on two weeks later. He wrote, "On the day after my surgery, at the doc's office, I tested 20/20 at distance vision and J-2 (the equivalent of 5-point font, like a small-print Bible) at near. That is the same as I tested after the surgery on my first eye. At the same appointment, my first eye (then two weeks after surgery) tested 20/20 at distance vision and had improved to J-1 (the equivalent of 4-point font, like mail-order catalogs) at near vision. I am euphoric."

I do want to mention that Bob had to spend extra money out of pocket to have multifocal intraocular lenses (IOL) implanted, as the majority of insurances only cover the basic monofocal IOL. There are several brands of multifocal IOL with different designs and various outcomes.

Besides multifocal IOL, other options include: monofocal IOL for distance and wearing reading glasses for near; monofocal IOL with monovision fit (one eye for distance and one eye for near); or one eye with multifocal IOL and

YOUR PRECIOUS SIGHT

another with monofocal IOL.

When I refer my patients to the surgeon for a cataract evacuation, I urge them to discuss the pros and cons of each option clearly with the surgeon, ask questions, and gather as much information as available to make a prudent decision.

We are talking about operating on your EYES! It's not like going to a barbershop to get a haircut or to a nail salon to get a manicure done.

~ * ~

The risk factors for adult cataracts are aging, diabetes, UV light, smoking, being overweight, hypertension (high blood pressure), history of eye injury or inflammation, history of eye surgery, systemic medication like steroids or for cholesterol (inconclusive), and other eye diseases.

The potential cataract surgery complications are intraocular lens dislocation, eye inflammation or infection, macular edema (swelling), ptosis (droopy eyelid), ocular hypertension, retinal detachment, increase number of floaters, posterior capsule opacification (PCO), corneal edema, increased light sensitivity, and seeing halos or starbursts at night.

For more information, please check out the References section at the back, under Chapter 20.

~ * ~

In my years of practice, I encountered several cases of congenital cataracts. A report indicates that about 0.4 percent of babies (four out of every one thousand) are found to have congenital cataracts at or soon after birth. Most of congenital cataracts I dealt with were at the peripheral portion of the natural lens, with no surgery required, but follow-ups were necessary. Nonetheless, if the cataract was dense and affected the central vision, I referred the child to a pediatric eye surgeon at once to prevent the development of amblyopia. For more information about congenital cataracts, please check out the References section at the back under Chapter 20.

YOUR PRECIOUS SIGHT

Chapter Key Points:

- Cataract is the condition in which the natural lens of the eye becomes cloudy, opaque, or discolored. Most cataracts are age-related and progress slowly; however, cataracts can occur at any age, even in infants (congenital) and young adults.
- Signs and symptoms of cataracts include: blurred vision, difficulty seeing at night or in dim light, sensitivity to glare or seeing a halo around lights, double vision, colors seeming to faded, frequent changes in glasses or contact lenses prescription (tends to shift toward nearsightedness).
- Risk factors for cataracts include the following: aging, diabetes, UV light, smoking, hypertension (high blood pressure), being overweight, previous eye injury or surgery, prolonged use of corticosteroid or certain medications, excessive alcohol intake, and family history.
- Cataract surgery is the procedure to remove the cloudy or discolored natural lens and replace it with an artificial lens, called an intraocular lens (IOL).

- Cataract surgery is a safe procedure with an extremely high success rate. However, it's paramount to follow the preoperative and postoperative precautions and medication regimen to avoid complications.
- The potential cataract surgery complications are intraocular lens dislocation, eye inflammation or infection, macular edema (swelling), ptosis (droopy eyelid), ocular hypertension, retinal detachment, increasing the number of floaters, posterior capsule opacification (PCO), corneal edema, increased light sensitivity, and seeing halos or starbursts at night.

Chapter 21

"Please just fill out the form so I can drive."

The Stories of Renewing Driver's Licenses and Safe Driving

"A driver's eyesight is critical in preventing car crashes, because nearly all the sensory input you need to drive a car comes from visual cues. If your eyesight is diminished, so is your ability to drive safely. This is especially important to senior drivers.

That's why most states require motorists to undergo vision tests as part of the driver's license renewal process. Depending on where you live, you may have a vision test in person at a state licensing office or submit results of a vision test performed by an eye doctor."

~AAA

DR. EICHIN CHANG-LIM

AS I ENTERED the exam room, Mr. Lee, seventy-eight years old, was pacing the room. He flapped the DMV form in front of my nose before I had a chance to greet him properly. This was his first visit to our office.

"Please just fill out this form so I can keep my license." He wasn't hostile, but neither was he amiable. His faint, authoritative voice cracked.

"Sit down, please. Let's go through the exam first," I responded.

"I don't need the damn exam. Don't waste time. I'll pay you anyway." He raised his voice and became agitated. "Just fill out the form. I need to drive." With a wide stance, he stood in the middle of the room.

I faced him squarely and insisted I would not fill out the form unless I did the eye exam. I also let him know I would fill out the form accordingly afterward.

He cursed vehemently.

"If what I said displeases you, you're welcome to go somewhere else," I told him in a quiet, yet unrelenting, voice.

He plopped down on the exam chair.

YOUR PRECIOUS SIGHT

During the case history, I discovered he had just moved from Northern California to So-Cal to be with his elder sister. His grown-up children lived in another part of the country. He took medications for hypertension and depression.

Mr. Lee was alert through the entire process. He'd already had cataract surgeries and had intraocular lenses in both eyes. The digital fundus photography revealed a few drusen and a myopic crescent at the temporal border of the optic nerve disc in both eyes. A myopic crescent is a white or grayish-white crescentic area in the back of the eye located on the temporal side of the optic disc. It has a strong correlation to the degree of nearsightedness. The significant size of Mr. Lee's myopic crescent indicated that he could be quite nearsighted before cataract surgery. His best correctable vision was 20/40 for both eyes. He was scheduled to return with a driver for a dilated fundus exam to check his peripheral retina.

On his DMV form, I marked that he needed to have a complete eye exam annually to renew his license. In addition, I wrote, "no freeway driving and no night driving" on the form.

He was calmed down and reasonable by the end of the exam, so I communicated with him intellectually. I explained to him the reasons for his restricted driving.

"I want you to get home an hour before sunset, stick with right turns as much as you can, and do not drive on cloudy or rainy days. And no freeway driving! You don't want them to take away your license, right?" I said.

I handed him a pamphlet, "A Transportation Service for Senior Citizens," which I obtained from the community services department at city hall. "Just in case you and your sister need it."

Please check out the link under Chapter 21, in the References section at the back of this books, on how to help seniors drive safer and longer.

~ * ~

"If an individual clearly demonstrates that he or she can drive safely, it is still important for family and friends to continue monitoring the individual's driving behavior, as the individual's driving skills may decrease significantly in a short period

YOUR PRECIOUS SIGHT

of time. ***The objective of monitoring is to detect a problem before it becomes a crisis.*** *If there are any doubts about safety, the person with dementia should not be driving."*

~Family Caregiver Alliance

THE EXAM ROOM was eerily still when I walked in. An older woman sat on the exam chair, her head bent and her eyes closed. Two other women sat in the corner. One's eyes were shut as though she was meditating; the other had a *People* magazine open on her lap, but I wasn't sure whether her mind was connected with the page.

The undercurrent of distress was palpable, despite the purported calm.

"Hi. Long time no see," I said to the woman with the magazine in her lap. In the back of my head, I debated whether to call her Sophia or Sonia.

She must've detected my hesitation. "I'm Sophia," she said.

Sophia and Sonia were sisters. They looked alike. I'd known them since they were young and had always had a difficult time getting their names correct. Now, they both had silver hair.

Sonia opened her languid eyes, straightened her back, and gave me a feeble smile as she greeted me.

Sophia cut to the chase. "Mom is due for renewing her driver's license. I wanted Sonia to come with me."

"I drove in last night from Arizona," Sonia confirmed.

"Mom was diagnosed with dementia six months ago. We don't know whether she should drive anymore. She got lost a few times, and I had to go find her," Sophia explained. She lived near Disneyland, about a thirty-minute drive from where her mom lived.

"She told me she still wants to drive," Sonia cut in.

"What's our liability if mom gets into a car accident and hurts someone?" Sophia asked.

While I was mulling over the question, Silvia, the mother, woke up. I'd known her for as long as I could remember. I loved and admired this lady for her abundant energy and big heart. She had done a lot of charity work for the community.

YOUR PRECIOUS SIGHT

Silvia's husband passed away some years ago, and she insisted on staying in the same house, alone. "I want to die in my own bed, in the same house," she once told me. Her desire to stay in the same place where she and her husband had shared a roof for over forty years was unwavering.

At this particular moment, Silvia stared forward. She seemed to be oblivious to what was going on. It had been nearly a year since the last time I saw the woman. Age and illness had definitely taken a toll on her.

I engaged with her to arouse her to full awakening. I did the entire exam with her. She did all right, despite some hiccups. Her ocular prescription had not changed much from the previous visit. However, due to her diminished cognitive ability, I could not sign the DMV form for her to renew her driver's license.

I communicated my decision to the daughters. "I don't think your mother should drive. Perhaps you should ask her attending neurologist for a second opinion."

"Silvia, let's not drive anymore. It's not safe for you," I said to the woman, reaching out to hold her hand and looking right into her eyes.

"I know," she murmured, tears shimmering in her gray eyes. "Thank you." She was trying to sound upbeat, but a tremor in her voice betrayed her desperation.

A few months later, Sophia brought her grandson in for an eye exam.

"Mom moved to Arizona. We found a nice nursing home near Sonia's place. Thank you for telling her not to drive."

"I'm glad everything worked out. Please give her my best," I said.

I consider it a happy ending, all things considered!

~ * ~

Let me end this chapter by sharing with you this quote from the Centers for Disease Control and Prevention (National Center for Injury Prevention and Control).

"Do you or your loved ones have a plan to stay safe, mobile, and independent as you age? Many people make financial plans for retirement, but don't consider how to plan for potential mobility

YOUR PRECIOUS SIGHT

changes. The mobility planning tool can guide you to take action today to help keep yourself—or your loved ones—safe, mobile, and independent tomorrow."

~ CDC

For more information, please check out the References section at the back, under Chapter 21.

Chapter Key Points:

- When evaluating a person's safe-driving ability, there are several visual conditions that are taken into consideration:

    - central vision/visual acuity
    - peripheral vision (aka side vision, which is the field of view that extends outward from the central portion of the visual field)
    - night vision (seeing well not only under low lighting, but requires one to see low-contrast objects)
    - glare resistance (the extent to which the driver can still see critical objects and events while facing a steady source of glare)
    - glare recovery (the rapidity with which the driver's vision functioning returns to what it was before the glare was encountered)
    - judgment of distance
    - eye movements
    - visual perception (the processing of incoming visual information).

YOUR PRECIOUS SIGHT

- Common eye diseases related to aging are glaucoma, macular degeneration, and cataracts.
- The family or friend of a person who was diagnosed with dementia should monitor his or her driving behavior and skills closely. If there are any doubts about safety, the individual with dementia should not be driving.
- For seniors who drive, the objective is to detect a problem before it becomes a crisis.
- According to the CDC, mobility planning—a plan to stay safe, mobile, and independent as one ages—is as relevant as financial planning for retirement.
- There are alternatives for people who are unable to drive due to aging or physical restrictions. Check out the local community transportation service agents.

Acknowledgments

Looking back on the life journey I have traveled, I am indebted to a long list of people who have touched and shaped me with love, encouragement, and sometimes, provocation. Thank you from the bottom of my heart.

This book would not have existed without the patients who trusted me, and the friends and professional associates who unwaveringly supported and guided me. My heartfelt gratitude to you all.

Great thanks to my dear friends, classmates, and colleagues, who, without hesitation, gracefully read the very first draft of this manuscript at my request.

Enormous thanks, specifically to you who not only took precious time amid your busy schedules to read the first draft but also provided me with your candid, invaluable feedback, which undoubtedly raised the bar and pushed this book to a higher caliber.

Thank you...

Alejandro M. Arredondo, OD, private practice

Bob Boyd, JD, attorney (retired), business advisor, speaker, and author of *Gone Camping*

Yao-Tseng Chen, MD, PhD, pathology specialist, Professor, Weill Cornell Medicine Physician

John Dolan, JD, attorney (retired) and author of mystery thrillers, including the *Time, Blood and Karma series* and *Karma's Children series*

Michael J. Jones, OD, private practice (retired)

John E. Larcabal, OD, private practice, Assistant Professor, Marshall B. Ketchum University, Southern California College of Optometry

Kenneth Lay, OD, private practice

Andrew R. Lim, OD, private practice

Dennis Lowman, OD, private practice

John H. Nishimoto, OD, MBA, FAAO, Professor, Senior Associate Dean for Professional Affairs and Clinical Education, Marshall B. Ketchum University, Southern California College of Optometry

Manling Sung, a kind friend whose endearing friendship spans over forty years

Suaree Torres, OD, group practice associate

Jane S.C. Tsai, PhD, PMP, FAACC, SVP International Affairs, YFY Biotech Management Company

Deepest thanks to my husband and two children. You have been there through the thirty-odd years of my full-time career as an optometrist and as a wife and a mother. You are my emotional partners partaking in the writing of this book.

Last but not least, many thanks to my editor, Susan Hughes. You always know how to correct my grammatical errors, adjust the wording, and polish the sentence structure to enhance the meaning of the text without distorting the intended content. You make my manuscript shine! I am so grateful for knowing you.

Three Kinds of Eye Care Professionals

Ophthalmologists

Ophthalmologists are medical doctors who provide full eye care, such as giving you a complete eye exam, prescribing corrective lenses, diagnosing and treating complex eye diseases, and performing eye surgery.

Optometrists

Optometrists are the primary eye care physicians, who provide many of the same services as ophthalmologists, such as evaluating your vision, prescribing corrective lenses, and diagnosing and treating eye disorders with drugs or selective surgical procedures. If it is needed, your doctor will refer you to a specialist accordingly.

Opticians

Opticians fill prescriptions for eyeglasses, including assembling, fitting and selling them. Some opticians also sell contact lenses, but only if the patient presents an updated and valid contact lens prescription from an OD or MD. However, opticians cannot perform eye exams in the United States.

Glossary of Common Eye and Vision Conditions

Astigmatism

A vision condition that causes blurred vision due either to the irregular shape of the cornea (the clear front cover of the eye) or sometimes the curvature of the lens inside the eye.

Blepharitis

An inflammation of the eyelids and eyelashes causing red, irritated, itchy eyelids and dandruff-like scales on eyelashes.

Cataract

A cloudy or opaque area in the normally clear lens of the eye, located behind the iris.

Color Vision Deficiency

The inability to distinguish certain shades of color. The term "color blindness" is also used to describe this visual condition, but very few people are completely color blind.

Computer Vision Syndrome

A group of eye and vision-related problems that result from prolonged computer use.

Conjunctivitis

A swelling or inflammation of the conjunctiva, the thin, transparent layer of tissue that lines the inner surface of the eyelid and covers the white part of the eye; may or may not be infectious.

Crossed Eyes

(Strabismus) - A condition in which both eyes do not look at the same place at the same time; usually occurs in people who have poor eye muscle control or are very farsighted.

Diabetic Retinopathy

A condition occurring in people with diabetes; causes progressive damage to the retina, the light-sensitive lining at the back of the eye.

Dry Eye

A condition in which there are insufficient tears to lubricate and nourish the eye.

Eye Coordination

Eye coordination is the ability of both eyes to work together as a team. Each of your eyes sees a slightly different image. Your brain, by a process called fusion, blends these two images into one three-dimensional picture. Good eye coordination keeps the eyes in proper alignment. Poor eye coordination results from a lack of adequate vision development or improperly developed eye muscle control.

Farsightedness (Hyperopia)

A vision condition in which distant objects are seen clearly, but close objects are blurred.

Floaters & Spots

The shadowy images that appear in the field of vision caused by particles floating in the fluid that fills the inside of the eye.

Glaucoma

A group of disorders leading to progressive damage to the optic nerve; characterized by loss of nerve tissue that results in vision loss.

Hordeolum (Sty)

An infection of an oil gland in the eyelid.

Keratitis

An inflammation or swelling of the cornea, the clear front cover of the eye.

Keratoconus

An eye disorder causing progressive thinning and bulging of the cornea, the clear front cover of the eye.

Lazy Eye (Amblyopia)

The loss or lack of development of clear vision in just one eye, not due to eye health problems; Eyeglasses or contact lenses can't fully correct the reduced vision caused by lazy eye.

Learning-related Vision Problems

Vision disorders that interfere with reading and learning.

Macular Degeneration

An eye disease affecting the macula (the center of the light-sensitive retina at the back of the eye), causing loss of central vision.

Migraine with Aura

A type of severe headache accompanied by various visual symptoms.

Nearsightedness (Myopia)

A condition in which close objects are seen clearly, but objects farther away are blurred.

Nystagmus

A vision condition in which the eyes make repetitive, uncontrolled movements, often resulting in reduced vision.

Ocular Allergies

The abnormal response of sensitive eyes to contact with allergens and other irritating substances.

Ocular Hypertension

An increase in the pressure inside the eye above the range considered normal without any detectable changes in vision or damage to the structures of the eye.

Pinguecula

An abnormal growth of tissue on the conjunctiva, the clear membrane that covers the white of the eye.

Presbyopia

An age-related vision condition in which the eye gradually loses the ability to focus on near objects.

Pterygium

An abnormal growth of tissue on the conjunctiva (the clear membrane that covers the white of the eye) and the adjacent cornea (the clear front surface of the eye).

Retinal Detachment

A tearing or separation of the retina (the

light-sensitive lining at the back of the eye) from the underlying tissue

Retinitis Pigmentosa

A group of inherited disorders of the retina (the light-sensitive lining at the back of the eye), which cause poor night vision and a progressive loss of side vision.

Valuable Resources

All About Vision

https://www.allaboutvision.com/conditions

American Academy of Ophthalmology (AAO)

https://www.aao.org/eye-health/a-z

American Optometric Association (AOA)

https://www.aoa.org/patients-and-public/eye-and-vision-problems/glossary-of-eye-and-vision-conditions

National Eye Institute (NEI)

https://nei.nih.gov/health

References

WHAT IS A DILATED FUNDUS EXAMINATION?

Animation: Dilated Eye Exam, National Eye Institute, NIH

https://www.youtube.com/watch?v=M6IlOKXlCqs&feature=youtu.be

CHAPTER 1

Lazy eye: Protect your child from amblyopia

https://www.allaboutvision.com/conditions/amblyopia.htm

CHAPTER 2

Color Vision Deficiency from American Optometric Association

https://www.aoa.org/patients-and-public/eye-and-vision-problems/glossary-of-eye-and-vision-conditions/color-deficiency

CHAPTER 3

Healthy Contact Lens Wear & Care by Centers for Disease Control and Prevention

https://www.cdc.gov/contactlenses/index.html

Contact Lenses and Cosmetics

https://www.aoa.org/patients-and-public/caring-for-your-vision/contact-lenses/contact-lenses-and-cosmetics

CHAPTER 4

The Eye and STIs

https://opto.ca/health-library/the-eye-and-stis

CHAPTER 6

Support Groups and Other Resources by Vision Aware

https://www.visionaware.org/section.aspx?SectionID=64&DocumentID=3222&rewrite=0

Resources for Parents of Children Who Are Blind or Visually Impaired

http://www.afb.org/info/living-with-vision-loss/familyconnect-8160/15

Living with Low Vision

http://www.lowvisioninfo.org/living.htm

Summary of the HIPAA Privacy Rule

https://www.hhs.gov/hipaa/for-professionals/privacy/laws-regulations/index.html

CHAPTER 7

Eye protection for sports: How to choose sports goggles

https://www.allaboutvision.com/sports/protection.htm

Tips for Selecting the Right Sport Protective Eyewear for your Child

https://www.libertysport.com/viewpoint/tips-for-selecting-the-right-sport-protective-eye-wear-for-your-child

UV and sunglasses: How to protect your eyes

https://www.allaboutvision.com/sunglasses/spf.htm

CHAPTER 8

LASIK surgery: Is it right for you?

https://www.mayoclinic.org/tests-procedures/lasik-eye-surgery/in-depth/lasik-surgery/art-20045751

Surgery for Refractive Errors

https://www.merckmanuals.com/home/eye-disorders/refractive-disorders/surgery-for-refractive-errors

CHAPTER 9

How Does an Early MS Diagnosis Impact Quality of Life?

https://health.usnews.com/health-care/patient-advice/articles/2017-04-07/how-does-an-early-ms-diagnosis-impact-quality-of-life?context=amp

Join a Local Support Group

https://www.nationalmssociety.org/Resources-Support/Find-Support/Join-a-Local-Support-Group

The MS Focus Independent Support Group Network

https://msfocus.org/Get-Help/Support-Groups.aspx

All Groups from the MS Connection

https://www.msconnection.org/Groups

CHAPTER 10

Central Serous Chorioretinopathy

https://www.asrs.org/patients/retinal-diseases/21/central-serous-chorioretinopathy

Conversion disorder: What you need to know

https://www.medicalnewstoday.com/articles/320587.php

CHAPTER 11

Chalk it Up to Drug Use?

https://www.reviewofoptometry.com/article/chalk-it-up-to-drug-use

Ocular manifestations of drug and alcohol abuse from the US National Library of Medicine

https://www.ncbi.nlm.nih.gov/pmc/articles/PMC4545665/

Smoking Can Lead to Vision Loss or Blindness

https://www.health.ny.gov/prevention/tobacco_control/docs/smoking_can_lead_to_vision_loss_or_blindness.pdf

Get Ready for Plain Packaging by the World Health Organization

https://apps.who.int/iris/bitstream/handle/10665/206456/WHO_NMH_PND_16.1_eng.pdf;jsessionid=

626266272322A86A60B51FC7293C9D75?sequence=1

CHAPTER 13

Pseudotumor Cerebri

https://www.hopkinsmedicine.org/healthlibrary/conditions/nervous_system_disorders/pseudotumor_cerebri_134,57

CHAPTER 14

Facts About Diabetic Eye Disease

https://nei.nih.gov/health/diabetic/retinopathy

CHAPTER 15

A consumer guide to bifocal and multifocal contact lenses

https://www.allaboutvision.com/contacts/bifocals.htm

CHAPTER 16

Do-It-Yourself Eyelid Scrub for Itchy Eyes

https://www.verywellhealth.com/autologous-serum-eye-drops-3422030

CHAPTER 17

Facts About Glaucoma

https://nei.nih.gov/health/glaucoma/glaucoma_facts

CHAPTER 18

Macular Pucker

https://nei.nih.gov/health/pucker/pucker

CHAPTER 19

Amsler Chart to Test Your Sight

https://www.macular.org/amsler-chart

What the Age-Related Eye Disease Studies Mean for You by NEI

https://nei.nih.gov/areds2/PatientFAQ

Facts About Age-Related Macular Degeneration

https://nei.nih.gov/health/maculardegen/armd_facts

CHAPTER 20

Facts About Cataract

https://nei.nih.gov/health/cataract/cataract_facts

Congenital cataracts: Causes, types and treatment

https://www.allaboutvision.com/conditions/congenital-cataracts.htm

CHAPTER 21

Vision by Senior Driving AAA.com

https://seniordriving.aaa.com/understanding-mind-body-changes/vision/

GLOSSARY

Glossary of Common Eye & Vision Conditions

https://www.aoa.org/patients-and-public/eye-

and-vision-problems/glossary-of-eye-and-vision-conditions

VISION TERMS

Key Definitions of Statistical Terms

https://www.afb.org/research-and-initiatives/statistics/key-definitions-statistical-terms

About the Author

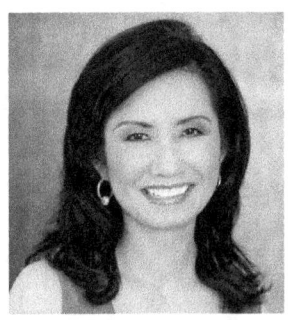

Dr. Eichin Chang-Lim is a semiretired optometrist, a multi-award-winning author, a wife, and a mother to 2 children. She and her husband had a private optometry practice in Los Angeles. They live in Orange County, California.

www.eichinchanglim.com

Twitter: @EichinChangLim

Facebook: @authoreichinchanglim

BookBub: https://www.bookbub.com/profile/eichin-chang-lim

www.ingramcontent.com/pod-product-compliance
Lightning Source LLC
Chambersburg PA
CBHW070618220526
45466CB00001B/39